Praise for The Mindful Way through Depression

"This is the book to turn to if you want to learn new ways to meet depression. It seamlessly weaves the science and practice of changing how we greet experiences, even profoundly difficult ones."
—J. DAVID CRESWELL, PHD,
William S. Dietrich II Professor of Psychology
and Neuroscience, Carnegie Mellon University

"An essential resource for anyone who struggles with depression. With clarity and compassionate understanding, the authors artfully combine the latest research with decades of clinical wisdom to offer an effective path forward. Filled with immediately relatable examples and easy-to-follow exercises, this book can help you not only to become freer from suffering, but also, ultimately, to live a richer life."
—RONALD D. SIEGEL, PSYD, author
of *The Extraordinary Gift of Being Ordinary*

"In this wonderful second edition, the authors once again seamlessly weave scientifically proven mindfulness techniques with insightful, compassionate stories. This book gives readers a completely new way to work with difficult emotions and thoughts. I can't recommend it highly enough!"
—LINDA E. CARLSON, PHD, RPSYCH, coauthor
of *Mindfulness-Based Cancer Recovery*

"Composed by a star-studded team of scientists and practitioners, this powerful book is the best self-help title to arrive since David Burns's seminal *Feeling Good*. . . . Highly recommended. (starred review)"
—*Library Journal*

The Mindful Way through Depression

Also Available

The Mindful Way Workbook: An 8-Week Program
to Free Yourself from Depression and Emotional Distress
John Teasdale, Mark Williams, and Zindel Segal

Mindfulness-Based Cognitive Therapy for Depression,
Second Edition
Zindel Segal, Mark Williams, and John Teasdale

Mindfulness-Based Cognitive Therapy
with People at Risk of Suicide
*Mark Williams, Melanie Fennell, Thorsten Barnhofer,
Rebecca Crane, and Sarah Silverton*

What Happens in Mindfulness:
Inner Awakening and Embodied Cognition
John Teasdale

the mindful way through depression

FREEING YOURSELF FROM CHRONIC UNHAPPINESS

second edition

Mark Williams, DPhil

John Teasdale, PhD

Zindel Segal, PhD

Jon Kabat-Zinn, PhD

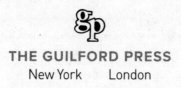

THE GUILFORD PRESS

New York   London

The information in this volume is not intended as a substitute for consultation with healthcare professionals. Each individual's health concerns should be evaluated by a qualified professional.

Purchasers of this book have permission to copy the Pleasant Events Calendar and the Unpleasant Events Calendar for personal use or use with clients. These worksheets may be copied from the book or accessed directly from the publisher's website, but may not be stored on or distributed from intranet sites, internet sites, or file-sharing sites, or made available for resale. No other part of this book may be reproduced, translated, stored in a retrieval system, or transmitted, in any form or by any means, electronic, mechanical, photocopying, microfilming, recording, or otherwise, without written permission from the publisher.

The vignettes in this book are composites of individuals we have known and are thoroughly disguised to protect individuals' privacy.

See page 262 for terms of use for audio files.

Printed in the United States of America

This book is printed on acid-free paper.

Last digit is print number: 9   8   7   6   5   4   3   2   1

Library of Congress Cataloging-in-Publication Data

Names: Williams, J. Mark G, author. | Teasdale, John D., author. | Segal, Zindel V., 1956– author. | Kabat-Zinn, Jon, author.
Title: The mindful way through depression : freeing yourself from chronic unhappiness / Mark Williams, DPhil, John Teasdale, PhD, Zindel Segal, PhD, Jon Kabat-Zinn, PhD.
Description: Second edition. | New York : The Guilford Press, [2025] | Includes bibliographical references and index.
Identifiers: LCCN 2024031695 | ISBN 9781462555512 (hardcover) | ISBN 9781462553921 (paperback)
Subjects: LCSH: Depression, Mental. | Happiness. | Attention. | BISAC: PSYCHOLOGY / Psychopathology / Depression | SOCIAL SCIENCE / Social Work
Classification: LCC BF575.H27 M56 2025 | DDC 616.85/2706—dc23/eng/20240805
LC record available at *https://lccn.loc.gov/2024031695*

Contents

Part IV
Reclaiming Your Life

Acknowledgments

This book would not have been possible without the considerable help and support of many to whom we owe an enormous debt of gratitude. We remain deeply grateful to those who read, and reread, the many earlier drafts of the first edition of this book for their help in clarifying the ideas we wished to express and for their suggestions on how best to express them: Jackie Teasdale, Trish Bartley, Ferris Urbanowski, Melanie Fennell, Phyllis Williams, and Lisa Morrison. We value greatly the professionalism and skills of all those at The Guilford Press who contributed to the production of the book, especially Barbara Watkins, Chris Benton, Kitty Moore, Anna Brackett, and Seymour Weingarten, and of those who contributed to the production of the audio recording, especially Dave Doherty at Soundscape Studio and Phyllis Williams. For this second edition, we are especially grateful to Kitty Moore and Chris Benton at The Guilford Press for their encouragement and advice. We gratefully acknowledge the help and support of our funders: the Wellcome Trust, the U.K. Medical Research Council, the Centre for Addiction and Mental Health (Clarke Division), and the U.S. National Institute of Mental Health.

It is a pleasure to thank all those fellow teachers and colleagues who over the years have supported and guided with their wisdom and knowledge the continuing development of our teaching of mindfulness, especially Christina Feldman, Ferris Urbanowski, Antonia Sumbundu, Helen Ma, John Peacock, and Chris Cullen.

Each of us owes a tremendous debt to our families, and especially to our wives, Phyllis, Jackie, Lisa, and Myla, for their love and unstinting support over the many ups and downs of bringing this project to fruition.

We also wish to thank the participants in our classes, who, through their courage, patience, and willingness to share their discoveries, have allowed us to make their experiences available to others through this book.

Finally, we are glad to have this chance to say that working together on this book has been a delight for each of us. In each other's company, in reading each other's words, in exploring each other's wisdom, we have discovered and valued again and again a deep resonance and a sense of an unfolding adventure shared.

■ ■ ■

The following publishers have generously given permission to reprint or adapt material from copyrighted works:

From "Cognitive Self-Statements in Depression" by Steven D. Hollon and Philip C. Kendall, in *Cognitive Therapy and Research, 4*, 383–395. Copyright © 1980 Springer Nature.

From "The Exhaustion Funnel" (unpublished work, 2004) by Marie Åsberg.

From *The Buddhist Path to Simplicity: Spiritual Practice for Everyday Life* (pp. 167 and 173) by Christina Feldman. Copyright © 2009 Christina Feldman. Reprinted by permission of HarperCollins Publishers Ltd.

From *The Sun My Heart: The Companion to the Miracle of Mindfulness* by Thich Nhat Hanh. Copyright © 2006 the Unified Buddhist Church, by permission of the Permissions Company on behalf of Parallax Press, Berkeley, California, *www.parallax.org.*

From *Collected Poems: 1945–1990* by R. S. Thomas. Copyright © 2001 Orion Publishing Group.

From *Mindfulness-Based Cognitive Therapy for Cancer* (pp. 144–145) by Trish Bartley. Copyright © 2012 Wiley-Blackwell.

From *Mindfulness: A Kindly Approach to Being with Cancer* (pp. 148–149) by Trish Bartley. Copyright © 2017 Wiley-Blackwell.

From *Letters to a Young Poet* by Rainer Maria Rilke, translated by Stephen Mitchell. Translation copyright © 1984 Stephen Mitchell, by permission of Random House, an imprint and division of Penguin Random House LLC. All rights reserved.

From "The Guest House" in *The Essential Rumi* by Coleman Barks, translated by J. Moyne. Copyright © 1997 Coleman Barks (Maypop Books).

From *The Poetry of Derek Walcott 1948–2013* by Derek Walcott, selected by Glyn Maxwell. Copyright © 2014 Derek Walcott. Reprinted by permission of Farrar, Straus and Giroux. All rights reserved. Reprinted by permission of Faber and Faber Ltd. (U.K. and Commonwealth rights).

From *The Mindful Way Workbook* by John Teasdale, Mark Williams, and Zindel Segal. Copyright © 2014 The Guilford Press.

Introduction

TIRED OF FEELING
SO BAD FOR SO LONG

Depression hurts. It's the "black dog" of the night that robs you of joy, the unquiet mind that keeps you awake. It's a noonday demon that only you can see, the darkness visible only to you.

If you've picked up this book, chances are you know these metaphors are no exaggeration. Anyone who has been visited by depression knows that it can cause debilitating anxiety, enormous personal dissatisfaction, and an empty feeling of despair. It can leave you feeling hopeless, listless, and worn down by the pervasive joylessness and disappointment associated with longing for a happiness never tasted.

We would do anything not to feel that way. Yet, ironically, nothing we do seems to help . . . at least not for long. For the sad fact of the matter is that once you have been depressed, it tends to return, even if you have been feeling better for months. If this has happened to you, or if you can't seem to find lasting happiness, you may end up feeling that you are not good enough, that you are a failure. Your thoughts may go round and round as you try to find a deeper meaning, to understand once and for all why you feel so bad. If you can't come up with a satisfactory answer, you might feel even more empty and desperate. Ultimately, you may become convinced that there is something fundamentally wrong with you.

But what if there is nothing "wrong" with you at all?

What if, like virtually everybody else who suffers repeatedly from depression, you have become a victim of your own very sensible, even heroic, efforts to free yourself—like someone pulled even deeper into quicksand by the struggling intended to get you out?

We wrote this book to help you understand how this happens and what you can do about it, by sharing scientific discoveries that offer a radically new understanding of what feeds depression or chronic unhappiness:

- At the very earliest stages in which mood starts to spiral downward, it is not the mood that does the damage, but how we react to it.
- Our habitual efforts to extricate ourselves, far from freeing us, actually keep us locked in the pain we're trying to escape.

In other words, nothing we *do* when we start to go down seems to help because trying to get rid of depression in the usual problem-solving way, trying to "fix" what's "wrong" with us, just digs us in deeper. The 3:00 A.M. obsessing over the state of our lives . . . the self-criticism for our "weakness" when we feel ourselves slipping into sadness . . . the desperate attempts to talk our hearts and bodies out of feeling the way they do—all are mental gyrations that lead nowhere but farther down. Anyone who has tossed and turned night after sleepless night or been distracted from everything else in life by endless brooding knows well how fruitless these efforts are. Yet we also know how easy it is to get trapped in these habits of the mind.

In the following pages—and in the accompanying audio recordings—we offer a series of practices that you can incorporate into your daily life to free you from the mental habits that keep you mired in unhappiness. This program, known as mindfulness-based cognitive therapy (MBCT), brings together the latest understandings of modern science and forms of meditation that have been shown to be clinically effective within mainstream medicine and psychology. The novel yet potent synthesis of these different ways of knowing the mind and the body can help you make a radical shift in your relationship to negative thoughts and feelings. Through this shift, you can find a way to break out of the downward spiral of mood so that it does not become depression.

Since we wrote the first edition of this book, the world has thrown up challenges that further exacerbate hopelessness and despair for many. These include our constant use of (and escape into) digital technology and social media that is a lifesaver for some but impairs well-being for others.

Then there are the deep existential fears and hopelessness brought on by world events like the COVID pandemic, drifts toward authoritarian politics, increasing disparity in wealth and privilege, ongoing racism, and the climate crisis. The extraordinary levels of turbulence created by these changes take their toll on individuals and families across the globe. While hopelessness and despair can seem a normal reaction to these situations, clinical depression makes things even worse: your low mood and self-blame undermine your energy and motivation just at the point when you need all the resources you can muster to cope with what's happening.

Mindfulness is not a quick fix or a Band-Aid to cover over the problems. It is a method that, little by little, opens up new ways of grounding yourself so that you may see what is going on in your inner and outer worlds more clearly. You begin to see how some understandable but habitual reactions can undermine your valiant attempts to help yourself and others. Millions of people have discovered that cultivating mindful awareness in the face of what is happening to them allows more spaciousness. They report a sense of open-hearted kindness in which the problems, still present, now feel more workable.

The promise that mindfulness can help people even in the midst of ongoing tragedy has motivated continuing research by ourselves and colleagues since the original publication of this book. Comprehensive reviews of data from worldwide studies of MBCT document a 31 percent relapse prevention advantage compared to usual care and show that MBCT is as effective at preventing new episodes of depression as antidepressant medication. We have found that the reduction in risk of relapse is even greater for those who have had the most severe and recurrent forms of depression associated with trauma during childhood and adolescence. We know more about who is most likely to suffer repeated bouts of depression, more about how mindfulness works to reduce risk, and how to sustain mindfulness practice in the long term. For example, neuroimaging has revealed that maintaining sensory awareness in the midst of sad moods—a core skill trained in MBCT—is associated with lowering the risk for depression's return, a theme we will return to in later chapters.

The women and men who have taken part in these studies had all suffered repeated bouts of clinical depression. But you don't have to have been officially diagnosed with depression to derive significant benefit from this book. Many people who suffer the hopelessness and pain associated with depression never seek professional help, but they still know they've been imprisoned by a chronic, persistent unhappiness that subsumes large stretches of their lives.

If you've felt yourself repeatedly floundering in the quicksand of despair, inertia, and sadness, our hope is that you will discover in this book something of potentially enormous value that can help you free yourself from the downward pull of low mood and bring a robust and genuine happiness into your life.

Exactly how you will experience the profoundly healthy shift in your relationship to negative moods and what will unfold for you in its aftermath are difficult to predict because they are different for everyone. The only way anyone can really know what benefits such an approach offers is to suspend judgment temporarily and engage in the process wholeheartedly over an extended period of time—in this case for eight weeks—and see what happens. This is exactly what we ask of the participants in our programs.

Along with the meditative practices, we will be encouraging you to experiment with cultivating attitudes of patience, compassion for yourself, open-mindedness, and gentle persistence. These qualities can aid in freeing you from the "gravitational pull" of depression by reminding you in key ways of what science has shown: it is actually okay to stop trying to *solve* the problem of feeling bad. In fact it is wise, because our habitual ways of solving problems almost invariably wind up making things worse.

As scientists and clinicians we came to a new understanding of what is and what is not effective in dealing with repeated depression by a somewhat circuitous route. Until the early 1970s, scientists had concentrated on finding effective treatments for acute depression—for that devastating first episode often triggered by a catastrophic event in one's life. They found them in the form of antidepressant medications, which remain enormously helpful in treating depression for many people. Then came the discovery that depression, once treated, often returns—and becomes more and more likely to recur the more often it is experienced. This changed our entire concept of depression and chronic unhappiness.

It turned out that antidepressant medications "fixed" depression, but only as long as people kept taking them. When they stopped, depression came back, even if not until months later. Neither patients nor doctors liked the idea of anyone taking lifelong medicine to keep the specter of depression from the door. So in the early 1990s we (Zindel Segal, Mark Williams, and John Teasdale) started exploring the possibility of developing an entirely new approach.

First, we set to work to discover what keeps depression coming back: what makes the quicksand more treacherous with every encounter. It turned out that every time a person gets depressed, the connections in the brain between mood, thoughts, the body, and behavior get stronger, making it easier for depression to be triggered again.

Next we started exploring what could be done about this ongoing risk. We knew that a psychological treatment called *cognitive therapy* had proven effective for acute depression and protected many people against relapse. But no one knew for sure how it worked. We needed to find out—not just out of theoretical interest but because the answer had huge practical implications.

Until that time, all therapies, both antidepressant medication and cognitive therapy, were prescribed to people only once they were already depressed. We reasoned that if we could identify the critical ingredient in cognitive therapy, we might be able to teach those skills to people *when they were well*. Rather than waiting for the catastrophe of the next episode to happen, we could, we hoped, train people to use these skills to nip it in the bud and prevent it from happening altogether.

Our individual lines of research and inquiry ultimately led us to examine the clinical use of meditative practices. We were interested in those practices that aim to cultivate a particular form of compassionate awareness, known as *mindfulness*, which originated in the wisdom traditions of Asia. These practices, which have been part of Buddhist culture for millennia, had been honed and refined for use in a modern medical setting by Jon Kabat-Zinn and his colleagues at the University of Massachusetts Medical School. Dr. Kabat-Zinn had founded a stress-reduction program there in 1979, developing an approach known as MBSR, or *mindfulness-based stress reduction*, which is anchored in mindfulness meditation practices and their applications to stress, pain, and chronic illness. Over the decades since then, MBSR, and programs based on it, have proved to be enormously empowering for patients with chronic diseases and debilitating conditions, as well as for psychological problems that arise from illness, pain, and trauma. These benefits have been confirmed not only in changes in the way people feel, think, and behave, and in clinical symptoms, but also in changes in the patterns of brain activity that underlie negative emotions.

Given how well-known mindfulness has become in the past few years, it is hard to recall that at first we had many doubts about what our colleagues and patients might say if we suggested using meditation as a preventive approach to depression. Nevertheless, the case for exploring whether Jon's work with MBSR could be adapted for depression was so compelling, we decided to take a closer look. The initial development of MBCT in the 1990s and the early studies and replications in the early 2000s that we described in the first edition have been followed by independent international studies that have established the effectiveness of MBCT. Since then this book has helped to disseminate MBCT across the world: it has been translated into twenty-three languages, and mindfulness teachers have been trained to teach it across almost every country. The MBCT manual (*Mindfulness-Based Cognitive Therapy for Depression*) has been published in an expanded *second edition* (2013), and MBCT has taken its place alongside the best evidence-based psychological treatment approaches for the prevention and treatment of major depression. We have also written *The Mindful Way Workbook* (2014) for those who have major depression but may not be accessing health services or who want to use self-help as an adjunct to professional help. Providing a highly accessible structured format of MBCT for depression, use of the workbook has been found to be more effective than self-help cognitive therapy in alleviating current depression.

The positive results of multiple MBCT clinical trials have resulted in the implementation of MBCT by clinicians and health commissioners from many countries. Teams from Oxford and Toronto have delivered much of the international training to build capacity in countries where no established MBCT services existed, including China, the Philippines, Hong Kong, Brazil, Taiwan, Singapore, Japan, Czech Republic, India, Hungary, Uruguay, and Poland. Hong Kong, Taiwan, Brazil, Uruguay, and Singapore now have established self-sustaining centers. As a result of all of these developments, MBCT has been adopted in health systems around the world. MBCT has also been offered in prisons. In 2017–2018, the Oxford team adapted MBCT for inmates in a large London remand prison. As part of the same project, the team also trained staff from a number of prisons to deliver MBCT, to ensure sustainability in the future. In a similar project in Taiwan, four prisons have introduced MBCT, and by October 2020 the program had been taught to more than four hundred prisoners.

In the United Kingdom's National Health Service, MBCT is now being disseminated widely to ensure it is accessible to those in need through the Improving Access to Psychological Therapies (IAPT) program. Fifty percent of these IAPT services now have MBCT-trained staff. A team led by Oxford colleague Willem Kuyken showed that outcomes of MBCT in these "routine clinical practice" settings match those seen in research settings: almost half of those entering treatment with depression recovered, and 96 percent of those in remission sustained recovery.

The continuing evidence for the impact of MBCT encouraged the U.K. Parliament to start offering mindfulness training to parliamentarians and staff, which led to recommendations for bringing mindfulness into health services, education, the criminal justice system, and workplaces. These developments encouraged parliaments in the Netherlands, Ireland, Denmark, France, Estonia, Wales, Scotland, and Iceland to establish similar mindfulness initiatives.

How to Make the Best Use of This Book

The first edition of this book, written in 2007, aimed to explain how mindfulness can help prevent depression and to make MBCT practices available to people who might not have ready access to an in-person MBCT program. There are now more courses and teachers available, but the need for mindfulness has also increased. Depression is on the rise, especially in young people, and accelerated by the COVID pandemic. Given its established clinical effectiveness, there remains an urgent need to ensure that anyone who needs MBCT can have ready access to it. This second edition aims to continue this task and to do so in a way that takes account of new research: for example, one of the most important discoveries since the first edition was written is that MBCT is effective at not only preventing new episodes of depression but also reducing current depression. We also know that MBCT is effective not only when conducted face to face, but when delivered by online therapy systems as well. Furthermore, we now know that the meditation practice in the program is an essential element of its effectiveness.

It is remarkable how the combination of Western cognitive science and Eastern practices has turned out to be one of the most powerful ways to break the cycle of recurrent depression. Why is it so helpful?

When depression starts to pull us down, we often react, for very understandable reasons, by trying to get rid of our feelings by suppressing them or by trying to think our way out of them. We wind up going over and over what went wrong or how things are not the way we want them to be. This is completely understandable. The problem is that, in the process, we dredge up past regrets and conjure up future worries. In our heads, we try out this solution and that solution, and it doesn't take long for us to start feeling bad for failing to come up with a way to alleviate the painful emotions we're feeling. We get lost in comparisons of where we are versus where we want to be, soon living almost entirely in our heads. We become preoccupied. We lose touch with the world, with the people around us, even with those we most love and those who most love us. We deny ourselves the rich input of the full experience of living. It's no wonder that we get discouraged and feel that there is nothing we can do. But this is exactly where compassionate meditative awareness can play a huge role.

The mindfulness practices taught in this book can help you take a wholly different approach to the endless cycles of mental strategizing that increase your risk of getting depressed. In fact, they can help you disengage from this entire pattern of mental activity. In this second edition, we offer new perspectives from recent research on how to cultivate mindfulness to help you let go of both past regrets and worries about the future. New research shows how MBCT increases mental flexibility so that new options open up to you when, the moment before, you may have felt there was nothing you could do. This is critically important for those who become suicidal when they become depressed. Our research has found that when depression recurs, the most common feature of depression to return is feeling suicidal: if you have felt suicidal during a past episode of depression, you are very likely to feel suicidal if sad feelings return. Can mindfulness help to "uncouple" depressed mood from suicidal feelings? It can: our research found that MBCT prevents the normal unhappiness we all experience from spiraling down into suicidal despair.

Part I of this second edition examines how the mind, body, and emotions work together to compound and sustain depression and what this view emerging from new research tells us about how to break out of this vicious cycle. It brings into sharp relief how we are all prey to habit-driven patterns—of thinking, feeling, and doing—that curtail the joy inherent in living and our sense of possibilities. It gives credence to the increasingly widespread message that there is an unsuspected power in inhabiting the moment you're living in right now with full awareness.

Mindfulness helps us get back in touch with the full range of our inner and outer resources for learning, growing, and healing, resources we may not even believe we have. One vital inner resource we often ignore or take completely for granted, whether depressed or not, is the body itself. When we get lost in our thoughts, we pay very little attention to the physical sensations from our bodies. Recent research has shown that it's worse than this: depressed and ruminative states of mind can actively inhibit sensory pathways. This is a new and very important discovery. Sensations within the body can give us immediate feedback about what's going on in our emotional and mental state. Body sensations can also give us valuable support in our quest to free ourselves from depression: focusing on them not only keeps us out of the mental trap of leaning into the future or getting stuck in the past but can also transform the emotion itself.

Logic and the knowledge of the latest research findings can be persuasive, but they are not necessarily of practical use in and of themselves, in part because they tend to speak only to the head through thought and reasoning. So Part II invites you to experience for yourself what any of us may be missing when we get totally caught up and lost in our mental gyrations, aimed at "fixing" our state of unhappiness, and lose touch with other aspects of our being and our intelligence, including the power of mindfulness. At this point it may be just an abstraction, another concept, to contemplate what it might mean to cultivate mindful awareness of your own mind, body, and emotions. That is why this section is designed to help you develop your own practice of mindfulness and see for yourself how profoundly transforming and liberating it may be.

Part III will help you refine your practice and bring it to bear on the negative thoughts, feelings, physical sensations, and behaviors that come together to create the spiral that can change unhappiness into depression.

In this edition, we add suggestions arising from recent research and practice to help you cultivate mindful awareness in a way that can be even more grounded, open, and compassionate.

Part IV brings everything together into one unified strategy for living more fully and more effectively in the midst of all of life's challenges and, in particular, the specter of recurrent depression. We share new stories of people who have grown and changed by engaging in the mindfulness practices in the face of their histories of depression, and we offer a systematic and easy-to-implement eight-week program for putting together all the elements and practices described in the book in a practical way. It is our hope that reading the book and engaging in the practices themselves will put you in touch with your inherent capacity for both wisdom and healing in the most practical and doable ways.

There are multiple ways to derive benefit from this approach. There is no need to commit yourself right off the bat to doing the whole eight-week program, although the benefits of doing so could be enormous when the time is right for that kind of commitment. In fact, you don't even have to have a specific problem with depression to benefit profoundly from engaging in one or more of the mindfulness practices described here. The habitual and automatic patterns of mind we will be examining afflict virtually all of us until we learn to come to grips with them. You may want simply to learn more about your mind and your interior emotional landscape. In doing so, you may be naturally drawn by your own curiosity to experiment with some of the mindfulness practices, perhaps starting with those in Part II. This experimentation, in turn, may motivate you to launch yourself wholeheartedly into the eight-week program and see what happens.

Two words of caution before we go further. *First, the various meditative practices that we describe often take some time to reveal their full potential.* That is why they are called "practices." They require revisiting, returning to them over and over again with a spirit of openness and curiosity rather than forcing some outcome that you feel is important to justify your investment of time and energy. This is really a new kind of learning for most of us, but one that is well worth experimenting with. Everything we cover here is meant to support you in your efforts.

Second, if you are in the midst of an episode of clinical depression, you should feel free to undertake the program, but take it one step at a time, at your own pace. Although new research has found that MBCT can be helpful even when you are still depressed, if it feels too hard for you right now, then wait until you have gotten the necessary help in climbing out of the depths and are able to approach this new way of working with your thoughts and feelings, with your mind and spirit unburdened by the crushing weight of acute depression.

Whatever your starting point, we encourage you to practice the exercises and meditations described here and on the downloads with a combination of patience, self-compassion, persistence, and open-mindedness. We invite you to let go of the tendency we all have to try to force things to be a certain way and instead work with allowing them to be as they actually already are in each moment. As best you can, simply trust in your fundamental capacity for learning, growing, and healing as we go along through this process—and engage in the practices as if your life depended on them, which in many ways, literally and metaphorically, it surely does. The rest takes care of itself.

Part I

Mind, Body, and Emotion

One

"Oh No, Here I Go Again"

WHY UNHAPPINESS WON'T LET GO

Gaia was depressed and distracted. She'd felt bad before but never as bad as this. Not just downhearted and miserable but overwhelmingly so—utterly worthless. She had made an appointment later that day with her physician. Here she was again, listlessly sitting at her desk, searching on the web for anything that might help instead of working on her project. She clicked on a link to a page on depression. She knew what it'd say. She always felt these articles were talking about her: first signs when in her teens, feeling a failure and unable to focus on her work. Withdrawing from the world. Sleeping problems.

Gaia stared into space, recalling with a shudder the first time she felt like this when she was in ninth grade: those times she couldn't make it to school. And her heroic attempts to pull herself through. She seemed to get better for a while, but at college she reacted badly when a friend ghosted her, and she dropped again into a deep despair. That was twelve years ago. She'd survived again by shutting things out, looking longingly at others who all seemed to be getting on with their lives.

During one of her times of despair she'd gone to a doctor who'd recommended antidepressants. They seemed to help, so she'd taken them for a year then been on and off them ever since.

Now, here she was, planning to leave her desk early to get to a physician appointment she knew would end with another recommendation to go back on the meds. She didn't know whether they'd help. Sometimes they did; sometimes they didn't. All she knew was that this wasn't the life she'd hoped for herself. It couldn't go on like this. Her boss would notice the work wasn't getting done.

Since COVID things had gotten worse; the loneliness of working from home was getting to her. Things at work had never recovered—working from home most days of the week; the office space gone; occasional meetings arranged in unfamiliar rented spaces around the town. No downtime to chat with colleagues over coffee. No distinction between workplace and home space. A good night's sleep a distant memory.

Jim hadn't had any trouble sleeping. In fact, he just seemed to have a hard time being awake. There he was again, sitting in his car in the office parking lot, feeling the sheer weight of the day pinning him to his seat. His whole body felt leaden. It was all he could do just to unlatch his seat belt. And still he sat, immobile, stuck, unable to grab the door handle and just go to work.

Maybe if he mentally ran through his schedule for the day . . . that always got him moving, started the ball rolling. But not today. Every appointment, every meeting, each phone call he had to return made him swallow what felt like an iron ball, and, with each swallow, his mind wandered away from the day's agenda to the nagging question that seemed to be with him every morning:

"Why do I feel so bad? I've got everything most men could ask for—a loving partner, great kids, a secure job. . . . What's wrong with me? Why can't I pull myself together? And why is it always this way? Wen and the kids are sick to death of my feeling sorry for myself. They are not going to be able to put up with me much longer. If I could figure it out, things would be different. If I knew why I felt so rotten, I know I could solve the problem and just get on with life like everyone else. This is really stupid."

Gaia and Jim just want to be happy. Gaia will tell you she's had good times in her life. But they never seem to last. Something sends her into a tailspin, and events she might have shaken off when younger now seem to plunge her into despair before she knows what's hit her. Jim says he's had good times too—but he tends to describe them as periods marked more by the absence of pain than by the presence of joy. He has no idea what makes the dull ache recede or return. All he knows is that he can't put his finger on the last time he spent an evening laughing and joking with family or friends.

As visions of being unemployed swirl through Gaia's head, a deep fear of being unable to do what she needed to do for herself lurked around the edges of her mind. *Not again*, she thought with a sigh. Gaia wasn't sure she could take it anymore. She had known friends who had become suicidal when they found themselves unable to cope like this. Such thoughts and images intruded into her mind from time to time, but she dealt with them by distracting herself. Recently, her attempts to distract didn't seem to work so well. Should she tell the physician or not? She wasn't sure she wanted it on her file. How had it come to this?

Jim had never been diagnosed with depression—he had never even talked to his doctor about his bleak frame of mind or his persistently low moods. He was surviving, and everything in his life was fine; what right did he have to complain about it to anyone? He would just sit there in his car until something came to him that would move him to open that door and get going. He tried thinking about his garden and all the beautiful new tulips that would be sprouting up soon, but that just reminded him that he hadn't really done the fall cleanup adequately and he'd have a lot to do to get the yard ready now, a thought that exhausted him. He thought about his kids and his wife, but the idea of trying to participate in mealtime conversation that night just made him want to go to bed early, as he had last night. He had planned to get up early to finish what he'd left on his desk yesterday, but he just couldn't seem to wake up. Maybe he would just stay at the office till he finished the thing once and for all, even if he had to be there till midnight. . . .

Gaia has recurrent major depressive disorder. Jim may suffer from a sort of low-grade depression that is more a persistent state than an acute condition. The diagnosis doesn't matter that much. The problem for Gaia and Jim and many of the rest of us is that we want desperately to be happy but have no idea how to get there. Why do some of us end up feeling so low over and over? Why do some of us feel as if we're never really happy but just dragging ourselves through life, chronically down and discontented, tired and listless, with little interest in the things that used to give us pleasure and make life worthwhile?

For most of us, depression starts as a reaction to a tragedy or reversal in life. The events that are particularly likely to produce depression are losses, humiliations, and defeats that leave us feeling trapped by our circumstances. Gaia became depressed as a teen, when she felt she'd lost her friends from middle school; she couldn't focus on the work and she didn't feel she fit in with any of the in-groups. In college she had barely survived, but since getting a job it was all she could do to take care of things when she returned from work at night, so she gave up postwork get-togethers with colleagues and shopping trips with her mother, and the texts to her sister became more and more rare. Soon she felt weighed down by loneliness, crushed by a constant sense of abandonment.

For Jim, the loss was a little more subtle and a lot less visible to the outside world. A few months after he received a promotion at his consulting firm, Jim found he no longer had time to spend with friends and had to drop out of his gardening club because he was staying later and later at the office. He also realized he didn't actually enjoy his new supervisory role. Eventually he asked to return to a job similar to the one he had done before. The change was a relief, and no one knew Jim wasn't happy—not even Jim at first. But he started getting spacey and seemed often distracted. In his head, Jim was second-guessing his decision, overanalyzing every brief interaction with his bosses, and ultimately chiding himself over and over for having "failed" his company and himself. He said nothing and tried to ignore these thoughts, but over the next five years he withdrew more and more, had a lot of minor health complaints, and, in the words of his wife, "just wasn't the man I used to know."

Loss is an unavoidable part of the human condition. Most of us find life an enormous struggle after the sort of episodes of depression that Gaia went through in her teens, and many of us feel diminished by disappointments in ourselves or others, as Jim did. But embedded in Gaia's and Jim's stories are clues to why only some of us suffer lasting effects from such difficult experiences.

When Unhappiness Turns into Depression . . . and Depression Won't Go Away

Depression is a huge burden affecting millions today and becoming more common in high-income as well as in low- and middle-income countries. Sixty years ago depression struck people first, on average, in their forties and fifties; today it's their early teens. Other statistics in the box below show the scope of the problem today, but none may be more alarming than the data showing that depression tends to return. At least 50 percent of those experiencing depression find that it comes back, despite the fact that they appeared to have made a full recovery. After a second or third episode, the risk of recurrence rises to approximately 80 percent. People who first became depressed before they were twenty years of age are at particularly high risk for becoming depressed again. What's going on here? As psychologists who had been involved in treating and researching depression for many years, three of us (Mark Williams, Zindel Segal, and John Teasdale)

THE PREVALENCE OF DEPRESSION TODAY

Around 12 percent of men and 20 percent of women will suffer major depression at some time in their lives.

The first episode of a major depression typically occurs between thirteen and fifteen years of age. Fifty percent of those who will get depressed experience their first episode before age eighteen.

At any one time, some 5 percent of the population are suffering depression of clinical severity.

Sometimes the depression persists; 15–39 percent of cases may still be clinically depressed one year after symptom onset, and 22 percent of cases remain depressed two years later.

Each episode of depression increases the chances that the person will experience another episode by 16 percent.

Ten million people in the United States are taking prescription antidepressants.

wanted to find out. The rest of this chapter, plus Chapter 2, explains what science has learned about the nature of depression and unhappiness and how that knowledge, once we banded together with our fourth author (Jon Kabat-Zinn), ultimately produced the treatment on which the first edition of this book was based, and which further study and research has developed.

One of the most critical facts we learned was that there is a difference between those of us who have experienced an episode of depression and those who have not: *depression forges a connection in the brain between sad mood and negative thoughts, so that even normal sadness can reawaken major negative thoughts.* This insight added a new dimension to our understanding of how depression works. Decades ago pioneering scientists like Aaron Beck had the insight that negative thoughts play a leading role in depression. Beck and his colleagues made a huge leap in our understanding of depression when they found that mood was strongly shaped by thoughts—that it wasn't necessarily events themselves that drove our emotions but our beliefs about or interpretations of those events. Now we know there is much more to the story. Not only can thoughts affect mood, but in those of us who get depressed, mood can affect thoughts in ways that can then make an already low mood even lower. It doesn't require a traumatic loss for those of us who are vulnerable to plunge down into the spiral again; even the kinds of everyday difficulties that many people shrug off can start the descent into depression or perpetuate unhappiness from day to day. Even more, as we'll see, this connection becomes so ingrained that sometimes the negative thoughts that lead to depression can be triggered by sadness so fleeting or minimal that the person experiencing it is hardly aware of it.

No wonder so many of us feel we can't pull ourselves out of the abyss, no matter how hard we try. We have no idea where the descent began.

Unfortunately, our valiant efforts to figure out how we got where we are turn out to be part of a complicated mechanism by which we get dragged down even farther. The way in which our efforts to understand ourselves can lead to additional problems instead of solutions is a complex story. It starts with a fundamental knowledge of the anatomy of depression and of its four key dimensions: feelings, thoughts, body sensations, and behaviors, through which we respond to the events of life. Key to this understanding is how these different dimensions interact.

The Anatomy of Depression

Let's look briefly at the development of the whole pattern of depression before we get into its individual elements.

When we become deeply unhappy or depressed, an avalanche of feelings, thoughts, physical sensations, and behaviors comes into play. Depression is more than sad mood. Our appetite changes: we may eat less and lose weight or find ourselves eating uncontrollably and gaining weight. Sleep is disturbed, and during the day it becomes hard to concentrate or think clearly. We may feel agitated, finding it hard to sit still; or we may slow down, finding it an immense effort to do anything. We lose interest in things we used to enjoy—as if someone has turned off our motivation switch. In the end, it can feel that life is just not worth living anymore, that we'd be better off dead; and we may find ourselves assailed by thoughts and images of how we could end this life. What's going on here?

The huge emotional upheaval that can come from experiencing loss, separation, rejection, or any reversal that brings a sense of humiliation or defeat is normal. Disturbing emotions are an important part of life. They signal to us and to others that we are severely distressed, that something untoward has happened in our lives. But sadness can give way to depression when the sadness turns into persistent harsh, negative thoughts and feelings. This morass of negative thinking then generates tension, aches, pains, fatigue, and turmoil. These, in turn, feed more negative thinking; the depression gets worse and worse and, with it, the hurt. We give up activities that normally nourish us, like getting together with friends and family. This only compounds our feelings of depletion by cutting ourselves off from those who might be a real support for us. Our exhaustion is compounded if we deal with it by simply working harder.

It's not difficult to see how feelings, thoughts, physical sensations, and behaviors are all part of depression. Earlier in this chapter we described the pain that Gaia felt as she sat at her desk mindlessly searching the internet, the "iron ball" that Jim felt like he had to keep swallowing when he thought about what his day held in store. As many of us are only too aware, being "down" can make it hard to do much of anything or to make choices that get us where we want to go. What's harder to see is how any one part of this anatomy can trigger the downward spiral and then how each component feeds into and reinforces the others. By this process the state of mind that keeps us unhappy or leaves us vulnerable to depression gets stronger and stronger. A closer look at the parts at this point may help us see the whole more clearly.

FEELINGS

If you think back to the last time you began to feel unhappy and describe your feelings, many different words might come to mind: sad, blue, down-hearted, miserable, despondent, low, feeling sorry for yourself. The strength of such feelings can vary; for example, we can feel anywhere from slightly sad to extremely sad. It's normal for emotions to come and go, but it is rare for such depressive feelings to occur by themselves. They often cluster with anxiety and fear, anger and irritability, hopelessness and despair. Irritability is a particularly common symptom of depression; when down, we may feel impatient, at the end of our rope with many of the people in our lives. We may be more prone than usual to angry outbursts. For some, especially young people, irritability is a more prominent experience than sadness in depression.

∞

The feelings by which we generally define depression are usually thought of as an end point. We're depressed; we feel sad, low, blue, miserable, despondent, desperate. But they're also a starting point: research has shown that the more we've been depressed in the past, the more sad mood will also bring with it feelings of low self-esteem and self-blame. Not only do we feel sad, we may also feel like failures, useless, unlovable, losers. These feelings trigger powerful self-critical thoughts: we turn on ourselves, perhaps berating ourselves for the emotion we are experiencing: This is dumb, why can't I just get over this and move on? *And, of course, thinking this way just drags us down further.*

∞

Such self-critical thoughts are extremely powerful and potentially toxic. Like our feelings, they can be both an end point and a starting point of depression.

THOUGHTS

Take a moment or two to imagine the following scene as vividly as possible. Taking your time, note, as best you can, what goes through your mind:

> You are walking along a familiar street. . . . You see someone you know on the other side of the street. . . . You smile and wave. . . . The person makes no response . . . just doesn't seem to notice you . . . walks right past without any sign of recognizing your existence.

> ▪ How does this make you feel?
> ▪ What thoughts or images go through your mind?

You may think there are obvious answers to these questions. But if you try this scenario on your friends and family, you'll probably get a range of reactions. What each of us feels depends critically on why we think the other person walked by us. This situation is ambiguous. It can be interpreted in a variety of ways and thus can evoke a range of emotional reactions.

Our emotional reactions depend on the story we tell ourselves, the running commentary in the mind that interprets the data we receive through our senses. If this scenario happens when we're in a good mood, the running commentary in our mind is likely to tell us that the person probably did not see us due to being preoccupied or not wearing their glasses. We might feel little or no emotional reaction.

If we're feeling a bit down that day, our story, our self-talk, may tell us that the person deliberately ignored us, that we've lost another friend. Our mind may spin off, ruminating about what we did to upset the person. Even if we had not been feeling very depressed at the start, this sort of self-talk can make us feel worse. If the self-talk says we've been ignored, we may feel angry. If it says we must have upset the person in some way, we may feel guilty. If it says we've probably lost a friend, we may feel lonely and sad.

Multiple different interpretations for the same set of facts are often possible. *Our world is like a silent film on which we each write our own commentary.* And different interpretations of what has *just* happened can affect what happens *next*. With a benign interpretation, we may quickly forget the incident. With a negative one, we may be pitched into the kind of self-chiding that Gaia did after realizing she'd been searching the internet again instead of getting on with work: *What's wrong with me? Why am I so useless? How long can I go on like this?* Negative thoughts often come in disguise, masquerading as questions that might have answers. Five or ten minutes later, the questions may still be nagging us, with no answers making an appearance.

Many situations are ambiguous, but the way we interpret them makes a huge difference in how we react. This is the A–B–C model of emotions. The A represents the facts of the situation—what a video camera would see and record. The B is the interpretation we give to a situation; this is the "running story" often just below the surface of awareness. It is often taken as fact. The C is our reaction: our emotions, body sensations, and behavior. Often we see the situation (A) and the reaction (C) but are unaware of the interpretation (B). We think the *situation* itself caused our emotional and physical reactions, when in fact it was our *interpretation* of the situation.

Gaia was sure her boss was sick of her. In actual fact, as Gaia would discover later, it turned out that her boss had been worried about her, but not, as she imagined, about the quality of her work, which, her boss said, had always been—and still was—amazing. Instead, her boss said that everyone on the team had suffered after the pandemic and with working from home, and she was concerned that Gaia might not be getting enough support for her work.

Jim was sure his family was sick of his self-pity and would soon reject him altogether. Actually, Jim's family was not sick of him at all, but really *worried* about him. They were desperate to come up with ways to cheer him up or just ignite a spark of life in him again. Jim was too ashamed of himself to take notice.

To complicate matters, our reactions then have an impact of their own. When we feel low, we're likely to pick out and elaborate on the most negative interpretation. Once we've seen someone pass us in the street and our low mood has brought to mind the interpretation that they "deliberately ignored me," this only makes us feel even lower. In turn, the increasingly deteriorating mood leads to questions about why this person "snubbed me," which only marshals more evidence to support our case of our own unlikability: *this happened to me just last week with so-and-so; I don't think anyone likes me; I just can't make lasting relationships; what's wrong with me?* The stream of thoughts begins to settle on a theme of worthlessness, isolation, and inadequacy.

If you're familiar with this kind of thought stream, it may be helpful to know that you're not alone in this pattern of negative thinking. In the box below you'll see a list of thoughts commonly expressed by depressed patients, compiled decades ago by psychologists Steven Hollon and Philip Kendall. The themes of worthlessness and self-blame permeate the list. If we're feeling okay at the moment, we might see quite clearly that these thoughts are distortions. But when we're depressed, they can seem like the absolute truth. It's as if depression is a war we wage against ourselves, and we marshal every bit of negative propaganda we can muster as ammunition. But who wins this war?

The fact that we often take these toxic and distorted thoughts about ourselves as unassailable truth only cements the connection between sad

---

AUTOMATIC THOUGHTS OF PEOPLE CURRENTLY DEPRESSED

1. I feel like I'm up against the world.
2. I'm no good.
3. Why can't I ever succeed?
4. No one understands me.
5. I've let people down.
6. I don't think I can go on.
7. I wish I were a better person.
8. I'm so weak.
9. My life's not going the way I want it to.
10. I'm so disappointed in myself.
11. Nothing feels good anymore.
12. I can't stand this anymore.
13. I can't get started.
14. What's wrong with me?
15. I wish I were somewhere else.
16. I can't get things together.
17. I hate myself.
18. I'm worthless.
19. I wish I could just disappear.
20. What's the matter with me?
21. I'm a loser.
22. My life is a mess.
23. I'm a failure.
24. I'll never make it.
25. I feel so helpless.
26. Something has to change.
27. There must be something wrong with me.
28. My future is bleak.
29. It's just not worth it.
30. I can't finish anything.

feelings and self-critical thought streams. Knowing this is vitally important to understanding why depression takes hold in some people and not in others or on some occasions and not on others. When such thoughts have affected us on one occasion, they remain ready to be triggered on other occasions. And when they are triggered, they drag our mood down even further, draining what little energy we have at a time when we need all our resources to cope with what has happened to us. Imagine what effect it would have on you if someone stood behind you all day telling you how useless you were when you were trying desperately to cope with a difficult experience. Now imagine how much worse it would be if the criticism and harsh judgment came from inside your own mind. No wonder it seems so real—after all, who knows us better than ourselves? These thoughts can trap us, turning a small sadness into a tangled web of brooding preoccupation.

∞

Negative thoughts can trigger depression or feed it once a low mood is upon us. We might sink into a glum mood by thinking Nothing ever goes right for me. *That mood may then trigger self-criticism like* Why am I such a loser? *As we try to unravel the cause of our unhappy state, our mood plunges. As we investigate questions about our worthlessness, we form a whole scheme of other negative thoughts, ready to be recruited at a moment's notice in the future.*

∞

Unhappiness itself is not the problem—it is an inherent and unavoidable part of being alive. Rather, it's the harshly negative views of ourselves that can be switched on by unhappy moods that entangle us. It is these views that transform passing sadness into persistent unhappiness and depression. Once these harsh, negative views of ourselves are activated, not only do they affect our mind; they also have profound effects on our body—and then the body in turn has profound effects on the mind and emotions.

DEPRESSION AND THE BODY

Depression affects the body, as demonstrated by the symptoms of major depression presented earlier. It rapidly leads to dysregulation of the body's rhythms. We might not feel like eating, which can eventually result in severe and unhealthy weight loss. Or we might overeat, gaining inordinate amounts of weight. Our sleep cycles can be disrupted in either direction too: either we feel low energy most of the time and sleep too much, or we find it difficult to get enough sleep. We may find ourselves waking in the middle of the night or early in the morning and being unable to get back to sleep. As in Gaia's case, we might churn over and over the events of our lives and the inadequacy of our response to them.

The bodily changes we experience in depression can have profound effects on how we feel and think about ourselves. If the changes in the body wind up activating old themes of how inadequate and worthless we are, then even minor and temporary changes in the body can make our low mood deepen and persist.

Eighty percent of those who suffer from depression consult their physician because of aches and pains in the body that they cannot explain. Much of this is linked to the tiredness and fatigue that come with depression. In general, when we encounter something negative, the body tends to tense up. Our evolutionary history has bequeathed us a body that will prepare for action when it perceives a threat in the environment, such as a tiger, that we need to avoid or escape from. Our heart rate speeds up, and blood is shifted away from the surface of the skin and the digestive tract to the large muscles of the extremities, which tense up in readiness to fight or flee or freeze. However, as we will see in more detail in Chapters 2 and 6, the most ancient parts of the brain make no distinction between the external threat of the tiger and internal "threats" such as worries about the future or memories from the past. When a negative thought or image arises in the mind, there will be a sense of contraction, tightening, or bracing in the body somewhere. It may be a frown, a stomach churning, a pallor in the skin, or a tension in the lower back—all part of a preparation to freeze, fight, or run.

Once the body reacts in this way to negative thoughts and images, it feeds back to the mind the information that we are threatened or upset. Research has shown that the state of our bodies affects the state of our minds without our having any awareness of it. In one study, psychologists asked people to watch cartoons and then rate how funny they were. Some of the people had to do this while holding a pencil between their teeth, so that they inadvertently tightened up the muscles used in smiling. Others had to hold a pencil between pursed lips, which kept them from smiling. Those who watched using their smiling muscles rated the cartoons as funnier. Another study asked people to watch cartoons while using frowning muscles. The inadvertent frowners rated cartoons as much less funny. In a third study, asking people to shake their heads or nod while listening to information influenced their judgments about the information. In all of these cases, the people involved were not aware of this physical influence.

What do these experiments tell us? When we're unhappy, the effect of that mood *on our body* can bias the way we evaluate and interpret things around us without our being even the slightest bit aware that this is happening.

Sam was driving home after a tough day at work. Eager to put it behind him, he looked forward to dinner and watching the basketball game on TV afterward. He had no idea that he had a white-knuckle grip on the steering wheel or that he had tensed his right arm muscles all the way up to his shoulder. But when a car pulled abruptly in front of him from a side street and forced him to put on his brakes, he leaned on the horn and yelled, "Idiot! You think you're the only one on the road?" He was surprised to feel his face grow hot, and suddenly he was grumbling mentally about the customer he'd had so much trouble with and how *that guy* thought he was the center of the universe too and how *no one* ever showed him any courtesy or respect and he was fed up with people messing up his job and everything else. By the time he got home, he'd lost his appetite, poured himself a stiff scotch, and refused to talk to his partner until the game was over.

∞

It's not just that patterns of negative thinking can affect our moods and our bodies. Feedback loops in the other direction, from the body to the mind, also play a critical role in the persistent return and deepening of unhappiness and dissatisfaction.

∞

The close links between the body and emotion mean that our bodies function as highly sensitive emotion detectors. They are giving us moment-to-moment readouts of our emotional state. Of course most of us aren't paying attention. We're too busy thinking. Many of us have been brought up to ignore the body in the interest of achieving whatever goals we are striving to attain. As a rule, we have not been taught to be attentive to our physical selves as a way of learning and growing, to enhance our effectiveness in social interactions, and even for healing. In fact, if we struggle with depression, we may feel a strong aversion to *any* signals that our body may be putting out. Those signals may be of a constant state of tension, exhaustion, and chaos in the body. We would prefer to have nothing to do with it in the hope that this interior turbulence will subside on its own.

Naturally, not wanting to deal with the aches, pains, and frowns means more avoidance and therefore more unconscious contraction in the body and the mind. Gradually, we slow down and are less and less able to function. Depression has started to affect the fourth aspect of our lives: our behavior.

DEPRESSION AND BEHAVIOR

As children or young adults, we may have been counseled by well-meaning people to "soldier on" or "just get over it" when we were feeling particularly downhearted or miserable. Perhaps, somewhere along the way, we picked up the message that it was shameful or weak to show our emotions. We naturally assumed that people would think the worst of us if they knew we were depressed.

The thinking that accompanies depression, with its core themes of inadequacy and unworthiness, is infinitely transportable to any situation. Without even knowing it, we can become stuck in believing with great certainty that virtually any stress or difficulty we experience is our fault and that it is our responsibility to sort it out for ourselves. And when working harder doesn't solve anything, that's our fault too. The result is overwhelming exhaustion.

Whenever Gaia's mood began to sink, and she felt her energy was just draining out of her, she consciously adopted a strategy of giving up her "unimportant" and "nonessential" leisure activities, which actually gave her pleasure, such as seeing friends or just going out for fun. As she saw it, this strategy made sense because it meant that she could focus her dwindling energies (which she viewed as a strictly limited fixed resource) on her more "important" and "essential" commitments and responsibilities. This is understandable, except that her essential commitments included meeting all the demands and expectations of family, friends, colleagues, and her boss, whether or not these were reasonable or realistic. In giving up the "unimportant" and "nonessential" leisure activities that might have lifted her mood and extended rather than depleted her reserves of energy, Gaia deprived herself of one of the simplest and most effective strategies for reversing a decline into depression.

Professor Marie Åsberg from the Karolinska Institute, Stockholm, has described this "giving up" as drifting down a funnel of exhaustion (see the diagram). The funnel is created when the circles of our lives become smaller and smaller. The narrower the funnel becomes, the more likely a person is to experience burnout or exhaustion.

Jim also had noticed that he no longer looked forward to seeing friends in the way that he normally did and that he wasn't getting the same kick out of the things that he used to enjoy. Each time he considered going out, the thought arose, *What's the point?—Nothing's going to make any difference to the way I feel, so I'll save myself the effort and stay in and rest—that will make*

THE EXHAUSTION FUNNEL

Sleep problems

Lack of energy

Aches and pains

Joylessness

Guilt

Depressed mood

Exhaustion

The narrowing area of the circles illustrates the narrowing of life as we give up the things in life that we enjoy but seem "optional." The result is that we stop doing activities that would nourish us, leaving only work or other stressors that often deplete our resources. Professor Marie Åsberg suggests that those of us who continue downward are likely to be those who are the most conscientious workers, those whose level of self-confidence is closely dependent on their performance at work, that is, those who are often seen as the best workers, not those seen as "lazy." The diagram also shows the sequence of accumulating "symptoms" experienced by Jim as the funnel narrowed and he became more and more exhausted.

me feel better. Unfortunately, as Jim was lying on the couch resting, his mind simply drifted into well-worn self-critical grooves. These, of course, all combined to create the perfect setup for the persistence and deepening of his depression. Jim's "rests" ended up making him feel even worse.

∞

Depression makes us behave differently, and our behavior can also feed depression. Depression certainly affects the choices we make regarding what to do and not do, and how to act. If we're convinced we're "no good" or unworthy, how likely are we to pursue the things that we value in life? And when we make choices informed by a depressive state of mind, they're more than likely to keep us stuck in our unhappiness.

∞

If we have been depressed before, a low mood can become easier and easier to trigger over time, because each time it returns, the thoughts, feelings, body sensations, and behaviors that accompany it form stronger and stronger connections to each other. Eventually, any one element can trigger depression by itself. A fleeting thought of failure can trigger a huge sense of fatigue. A small comment by a family member can trigger an avalanche of emotions such as guilt and regret, feeding a sense of inadequacy. Because these downward spirals are so easily triggered by small events or mood shifts, they feel as if they come out of nowhere. And once depression takes hold, we can feel powerless to prevent it from getting worse or to make it better. All our attempts to control our thoughts or to snap out of our feelings are to no avail, and a full-blown episode of depression may return. And our research on the psychological processes underlying vulnerability has revealed a hidden feature of such recurrent depression: how sad mood can reactivate suicidal ideas. Although most symptoms of depression vary from one episode of depression to the next, if we feel suicidal in one episode, then it's very likely we'll feel suicidal in the next as well. People who have reacted to relatively mild changes in mood with a large increase in suicidality find these thoughts coming back again and again. This gives us even more reason to find a way to prevent the next episode.

What can we do to prevent the normal and understandable emotion of unhappiness from persisting or spiraling down into depression? Our first challenge will be to understand why it is that we feel so powerless to change how we are feeling and why, despite valiant efforts to assert control, we are continually getting ourselves more and more stuck. As we stated in the Introduction, we will discover that there are very good reasons for this. It is not for want of trying or because there is actually something wrong with us. Rather, it is because our efforts have taken us in the wrong direction!

Freedom from depression is possible, but that freedom comes from an entirely different perspective and understanding of what the problem actually is. This new perspective will serve as a map to guide us into uncharted territory within our own being and experience, where we can tap into and harness deep interior resources of the mind that most of us never suspected we had.

Two

The Healing Power
of Awareness

MAKING A SHIFT TO FREEDOM

It's not our fault that we repeatedly get depressed. We start to feel bad, and before we know it we've been pulled down into the spiral, and no amount of struggle will get us out. In fact, the more we struggle, the deeper we end up mired. We may blame ourselves for feeling bad in the first place—and especially for feeling worse the more we think about it. But what is really at work is a certain mental pattern, or mode of mind, that is triggered so automatically by unpleasant emotion that we hardly notice or know what is actually happening.

To see these mental mechanisms for what they are, we have to explore emotion and how we react to it. This exploration will reveal exactly how the struggle itself pulls us down—and how unjust it is to blame ourselves. Even more important, understanding that it is a certain mode of mind that gets us stuck opens the door to an alternative way of dealing with emotion: making a radical shift to a different mode of mind. Within that very shift, practiced over and over again in key moments, lies the possibility of transforming our relationship with depression and freeing ourselves from its grip.

The Role of Emotion

On one important level, our emotions are vital messengers. They evolved as signals to help us meet our basic needs for self-preservation and safety and to survive individually and as a species. The human emotional repertoire is remarkably sophisticated, its inner and outer expressions and messages often eloquent and complex. Even so, there are really only a few basic families of emotions. The most prominent are happiness, sadness, fear, disgust, and anger, with each emotion having different ways of expressing itself. Each one is a full-body reaction to a characteristic situation: fear is triggered when danger threatens; sadness and grief when something precious is lost; disgust when something highly unpleasant is confronted; anger when an important goal is blocked; happiness when our needs are met. Naturally, we pay attention to these signals. They tell us what to do to survive and even thrive.

For the most part, our emotional reactions evolved to be temporary. They have to be. The messenger needs to be alert to the need to signal the next alarm. Our initial emotional reaction lasts only as long as the subject of the alarm continues—often a few seconds rather than a few minutes. For it to last longer would make us insensitive to further changes in the environment. We can see this clearly in the behavior of gazelle on the African savannah. Fear drives them to run desperately to avoid the predator that is chasing the herd. But once a gazelle has been captured, the rest of the herd rapidly resumes grazing, as if nothing had happened. The situation has changed; the danger is past; the herd also needs to eat to survive.

Of course, some situations endure, and so may our emotional reaction to them. Sadness as a response to the loss of someone dear to us may continue for a long time. Grief can continue to come in unexpected waves that may well up and overwhelm us for many weeks and months after the loss. Even here, however, the mind has ways of healing itself. Even with grief, most people find that, little by little, life eventually returns to some sense of normality and we begin to discover the possibility of smiling and laughing once again.

Why, then, do depression and unhappiness outlast the situations that trigger them? Or why, sometimes, does a sense of malaise and dissatisfaction go on and on? The short answer is that these emotions persist because we have emotional reactions to our own emotions that actually keep them going.

THE PROBLEM WITH OUR OWN EMOTIONAL REACTIONS TO OUR EMOTIONS

Carole often finds herself feeling "a little miserable" right before she goes to bed. Naturally this bothers her, especially because she can't always connect the feeling to any event that directly precedes the mood. "Last Friday, for example," she explained, "Angie came over and we spent the evening watching a film. Everything was fine. Then after she left, I went around the apartment clearing up, and I realized that a feeling of sadness had crept up on me. I started to think of times in the past when friends had let me down. When this happens, my mind always goes along the same lines: *Why am I feeling miserable again and dragging all this up?* Was I miserable all evening but just distracting myself because Angie was here, or is it the silence at bedtime that gets to me?"

Carole often tries to distract herself from her mood by sitting up in bed scrolling through her phone or channel-surfing the TV . . . but she finds that it doesn't help. She is soon distracted by her own thoughts.

"I try to find a reason why I'm feeling the way I am: *What happened today that made me feel like this?* I can usually think of something that went wrong, like when Jean went out for lunch without telling me she was going, and I wondered whether we are still friends. But it often doesn't really feel like it explains how I am feeling right now. So I start wondering what is wrong with me that I feel this way when other people seem quite happy. Soon I've dragged up lots of negative stuff, and I start to think, *Perhaps I'm always going to feel this way. How will my life be if these feelings last? How will I get on with people or do my job then? Will I ever feel really happy?* And, of course, that just drags me down further. I end up feeling really bad about myself: everything seems to take so much effort—making friends, doing my job, everything.

"Sometimes I can see exactly what I'm doing: I'm making myself more miserable. I say to myself: *All this thinking is doing me no good at all. So why do I do this to myself all the time?* Then I set off on another round of thinking about what's wrong with me."

Carole could see that her reactions to her sadness were actually making her more miserable. Her attempts to feel better—by trying desperately to understand what was going on in her mind—actually made her feel worse. Our reactions to unhappiness can transform what might otherwise be a brief, passing sadness into persistent dissatisfaction and unhappiness.

The problem with persistent and recurrent depression is not "getting sad" in the first place. Sadness is a natural mind-state, an inherent part of being human. It is neither realistic nor desirable to imagine that we can or should get rid of it. The problem is what happens next, immediately after the sadness comes.

"GET ME OUT OF HERE!"

The fact is that when emotions are telling us that something is not as it should be, the feeling is distinctly uncomfortable. It's meant to be. The signals are exquisitely designed to push us to act, to do something to rectify the situation. If the signal didn't feel uncomfortable, didn't create an urge to act, would we leap out of the path of a speeding truck, step in when we saw a child being bullied, turn away from something that we found repugnant? It's only when the mind registers that the situation is resolved that the signal shuts itself off.

When the problem that our emotions signal needs to be solved is "*out there*"—a charging bull or a roaring funnel cloud—reacting in a way that will allow us to avoid it or escape from it makes sense. The brain mobilizes a whole pattern of mostly automatic reactions that help us deal with whatever is threatening our survival, helping us get rid of or avoid the threat. We call this initial pattern of reactions—in which we feel negatively toward and want to avoid or eliminate something—*aversion*. Aversion forces us to act in some appropriate way to the situation and thereby turn off the warning signal. In this regard, it can serve us well, can even save our lives. Sometimes.

But it's not hard to see that the same reactions are going to be counterproductive and even dangerous to our well-being when directed at what's going on "*in here*"—toward our own thoughts, feelings, and sense of self.

None of us can run fast enough to escape our own inner experience. Nor can we eliminate unpleasant, oppressive, and threatening thoughts and feelings by fighting with them and trying to annihilate them.

When we react to our own negative thoughts and feelings with aversion, the brain circuitry involved in physical avoidance, submission, or defensive attack (the "avoidance system" of the brain) is activated. Once this mechanism is switched on, the body tenses as if it were either getting ready to run or bracing itself for an assault. We can also sense the effects of aversion in our minds. When we are preoccupied, dwelling on how to get rid of our feelings of sadness or disconnection, our whole experience is one of contraction. The mind, driven to focus on the compelling yet futile task of getting rid of these feelings, closes in on itself. And with it, our experience of life itself narrows. Somehow we feel cramped, boxed in. The choices available to us seem to dwindle. We come to feel increasingly cut off from the wider space of possibilities that we long to connect with.

Over our lifetime, we may have come to dislike or even hate emotions such as fear, sadness, or anger, in ourselves and in others. If we have, for example, been taught not to "be so emotional," we will have picked up the message that expression of emotion is somewhat unseemly and may have assumed it wasn't okay to *feel* emotion either. Or maybe we remember clearly the drawn-out feeling of an emotional experience like grief and now react with dread when a hint of similar feelings arises.

When we react negatively—with aversion—to our own negative emotions, treating them as enemies to be overcome, eradicated, and defeated, we get into trouble. So understanding aversion becomes fundamental to understanding what gets us stuck in persistent unhappiness. We run into problems because the unhappiness we are feeling *now* triggers old, extraordinarily unhelpful patterns of thinking from the *past*.

Mood and Memory

Have you ever visited a place that you haven't been to for many years, perhaps since childhood? Before the visit, memory of things that happened at that time of your life may be quite sketchy. But once you get there, walking down the streets, taking in the smells and the sounds may bring it all back—not just memories, but feelings: of excitement, of sorrow, of first love. Returning to the place—the old context—does something that our best efforts to remember could not do nearly as well.

Context has incredibly powerful effects on memory. Memory researchers Duncan Godden and Alan Baddeley found that if deep-sea divers tried to commit something to memory while on the beach, they tended to forget it when under water and were able to recall it fully only when they were back on dry land. It worked the other way around too. If they learned a list of words under water, their memory of that list when on dry land was not so good, but came back when they returned to the water. The sea and the beach acted as powerful contexts for the memory, just like a visit to a childhood town or an old campus haunt. Although this experiment is hard to repeat, other scientists have found a similar effect using virtual reality environments deliberately designed to be very distinct (for example an "underwater" versus a "Mars planet" environment).

MEMORIES TRIGGERED BY MOOD

Over the last few decades, psychologists have discovered something really important about how our emotional states can have such pervasive effects on our minds. A mood can function as an internal context; it can act in the same way that the sea did for the divers, bringing back memories and patterns of thinking that are associated with times when we were in that mood, just as if we had dived again into that particular stretch of water. *When we return to that mood, thoughts and memories related to whatever was going on in our mind or world to make us unhappy will come back quite automatically, whether we want it to happen or not.* When the mood comes up again, so do the thoughts and memories connected with it, *including the thinking patterns that created that mood.*

Because we live different lives, the experiences that provoked unhappiness in the past will differ from one person to another. For that reason, *we differ, one from another, in the kinds of memories and thinking patterns that get reactivated by the moods we are experiencing in this moment.* If the main things that made us sad in the past were losses, such as the sad but expected death of a beloved grandparent, when we feel passing sadness now, these will be the memories that come to mind. We may feel sad again, but we may have no trouble acknowledging our loss and then shifting the focus of the mind to other things while the echo of the grief fades in its own good time.

But what if our previous moods of unhappiness or depression were evoked by situations that somehow led to our thinking and feeling that we were not good enough, that we were worthless, or frauds? We saw (in the box on page 19) that a first episode of depression occurs most commonly between thirteen and fifteen years of age. Sadly, we now know that many people who become depressed as adults have experienced trauma, such as physical, emotional, or sexual abuse when they were children or adolescents. And even if such trauma did not occur, adolescence is a time when, without the life skills we now have, feelings of being a failure in comparison with others, of being lonely, or of being just plain no good can be overwhelming. If such experiences were a significant part of your childhood, the thinking patterns that made you depressed *then*, the sense that you are not good enough in some way, are highly likely to be reactivated in the present by even a passing feeling of depression.

∞

We can react so negatively to unhappiness because our experience is not one simply of sadness, but is colored powerfully by reawakened feelings of deficiency or inadequacy. What may make these reactivated thinking patterns most damaging is that we often don't realize they are memories at all. We feel not good enough now without being aware that it is a thinking pattern from the past that is evoking the feeling.

∞

When Carole was fourteen, she changed schools when her parents moved across the state. She missed her old friends, and although they had promised to stay in touch, it didn't happen. She found it really hard to make friends at her new school, and she deliberately kept to herself, not joining in activities with others, and soon they ignored her completely. She felt lonely, cut off, and unwanted.

Carole couldn't wait to get out of high school. She came back into her own in college. But she was always prey to unpredictable mood shifts that would drain her of energy and send her shuffling back into an isolated corner somewhere, sometimes for a few weeks at a time. Her mood could begin to slide at any time. Recently any slight sadness could retrigger the whole constellation of feelings of inadequacy from the past, leaving her feeling lonely and friendless. When this happened, she found herself unable to switch her attention back to what she was doing—her mind seemed completely taken over by her feelings.

Carole's experience shows clearly the cycle that afflicts so many people. Once negative memories, thoughts, and feelings, reactivated by unhappy moods, have forced their way into our consciousness, they produce two major effects. First, naturally enough, they increase our unhappiness, as Carole found, depressing mood even further. Second, they will bring with them a set of seemingly urgent priorities for what the mind has absolutely got to focus on—our deficiencies and what we can do about them. It is *these* priorities that dominate the mind and make it so difficult to switch attention to anything else. Thus we find ourselves compulsively trying over and over to get to the bottom of what is wrong with us as people, or with the way we live our lives, and fix it.

Caught up in this way, how on earth could we possibly contemplate switching our attention away from these pressing and understandable concerns to focus on other topics or approaches, even if doing so might contribute to a lightening of our mood? Sorting things out and forcing a solution will always seem like the most compelling thing to do—figuring out what it is that is not good enough about us, sorting out what we need to do to minimize the havoc that our unhappiness will wreak in our lives if it persists. But in fact focusing on these issues in this way is using exactly the wrong tools for the job. It simply fuels further unhappiness and keeps us fixated on the very thoughts and memories that are making us unhappy. It is as if a horror story were being enacted in front of us: we hate looking, but, at the same time, we can't turn away.

THE CRITICAL MOMENT

We can't change the fact that past memories and self-critical and judgmental ways of thinking are triggered when we feel unhappy. It all happens quite automatically. But we may be able to change what happens next.

If Carole had seen how a slight shift in her mood was reactivating *old* patterns of mind that were around at a time in her life when she felt alone, misunderstood, and devalued, she might have been able to let it float by and gone on with her day. She might even have been able to treat herself with a little kindness.

We *can* learn to relate differently to our unhappiness in just those ways. The first step is to see even more clearly the ways in which we entangle ourselves. In particular, we need to become more aware of the pattern, or mode, of mind that gets switched on and can cause so much suffering.

Doing Mode: When Critical Thinking Volunteers for a Job It Can't Do

When the thinking reawakened by depressed mood tells us that *we* are the problem, we want to get rid of these feelings *right now*. But larger issues have been triggered and dredged up: it is not just that *today* is not going well; our whole *life* feels as if it is not going well. We feel caught in a prison, and we *have* to find a way to escape.

The problem is that we try to think our way out of our moods by working out what's gone wrong. *What's wrong with me? Why do I always feel overwhelmed?* Before we have any idea what hit us, we're compulsively trying over and over to get to the bottom of what is wrong with us as people or with the way we live our lives, *and fix it*. We put all of our mental powers to work on the problem, and the power we rely on is that of our critical thinking skills.

Unfortunately, those critical thinking skills *might be exactly the wrong tools for the job*.

We're rightly proud of what we can do through critical analytical thinking. It's one of the highest achievements of our evolutionary history as human beings and does get us out of a whole slew of fixes in life. So when we see things are not going well in our *internal*, emotional life, it's hardly surprising that the mind often quickly reacts by recruiting the mode of mind that functions so effectively in solving problems in our *external* world. This mode of careful analysis, problem solving, judgment, and comparison is aimed at closing the gap between the way things are and the way we think they should be—at solving perceived problems. Therefore we call it the *doing mode of mind*. It's the mode by which we respond to what we hear as a call to action.

Doing mode is mobilized because it usually works very well in helping us achieve our goals in everyday situations and in solving work-related technical problems. Consider the simple everyday action of driving across town. For making a journey, the doing mode of mind enables us to reach the goal by creating an idea of where we are now (at home) and an idea of where we want to be (at the stadium). It then automatically focuses on the mismatch between these two ideas, generating actions aimed at narrowing the gap (get in the car and drive). It continuously monitors whether the gap is getting bigger or smaller to check whether these actions are having the desired effect of reducing the "distance left to travel" between the two ideas. If need be, it adjusts the actions to make sure the gap is decreasing rather than increasing. It then repeats the process over and over again. Finally, the gap is closed, we've reached our destination, the goal has been achieved, and the doing mode is ready to take on the next task.

This strategy offers us a very general approach for attaining our goals and solving our problems: if there is something we want to happen, we focus on narrowing the gap between our idea of where we are and our idea of where we want to be. If there is something we *don't* want to happen, we focus on increasing the gap between our idea of where we are and our idea of what we want to avoid. This doing mode of mind not only enables us to manage the routine details of our daily lives but also underlies some of the most awe-inspiring accomplishments of the human species in transforming the external world, from the construction of the pyramids to the engineering feat of modern skyscrapers. All these achievements required exquisite and elegant problem solving of a certain kind. It is quite natural, then, that the same mental strategies should get recruited when we want to transform our internal world—to change ourselves so that we can attain happiness, for example, or get rid of unhappiness. Unfortunately, this is where things can start to go horribly wrong.

WHY WE CAN'T PROBLEM-SOLVE OUR EMOTIONS

Imagine yourself walking along a path by a river on a sunny day. You're feeling a little down, a little out of sorts. At first you're not really aware of your mood, but then you realize you don't feel very happy. You're also aware that the sun is shining. You think, *It's a lovely day; I should be feeling happy.*

Let that thought sink in: *I should be feeling happy.*

How do you feel now? If you feel worse, you're not alone. Virtually everyone reports the same response. Why? Because, in the case of our moods, the very act of focusing on the gap, comparing how we are feeling with how we want to feel (or how we think we *should* feel), makes us feel unhappy, taking us even further away from how we want to be. Focusing on the gap in this way is actually a reflection of the mind's habitual strategy for trying to sort out situations in which things aren't as we want them to be.

Normally, if our mood is not too intense, we may hardly notice the slight downturn in our feelings when we make a comparison between how we feel and how we'd like to feel. However, if the mind is in doing mode—trying to solve "problems" like "What's wrong with me?" and "Why am I so weak?"—*we can get trapped in the very thinking that was recruited to rescue us.* This is *"driven-doing"*—the mind brings up (and then holds in consciousness) the relevant ideas it is working on—for instance, an idea of the kind of person I am right now (sad and lonely), an idea of the kind of person I want to be (peaceful and happy), and an idea of the kind of person I fear I might become if the sadness persists and I sink into depression (pathetic and weak). The driven-doing mode then relentlessly focuses on the mismatch between these ideas, the ways in which we are not the people we want to be.

Focusing on the mismatch between our idea of the people we want to be and our idea of the people we see ourselves as makes us feel worse than we did in the first place, when the doing mode started its attempts to help. It uses mental time travel to "help," calling up past times when we may have felt like this in an effort to understand what went wrong, and imagining a future, blighted by unhappiness, to remind us that this is what we desperately need to avoid. The memories of previous failures and the images of feared future scenarios that we bring to mind in the process add their own twist to the spiral of worsening mood. The more we have suffered low mood in the past, the more negative will be the images and self-talk unlocked by our present mood, and the more our mind will be dominated by these old patterns. But they seem real to us *now.* These patterns of feeling worthless or lonely feel familiar, but instead of seeing the feeling of familiarity as a sign that the mind is going down an old mental groove, *we take the feeling of familiarity to mean that it must all be true.* That's why we can't snap out of it, as our family and friends may have been urging. We cannot let go, because the "driven-doing" mind insists that our highest priority is to sort ourselves out by identifying and solving this "problem." So we hammer ourselves with more questions: "Why do I always react this way?," "Why can't I handle things better?," "Why do I have problems other people don't have?," "What am I doing to deserve this?"

You may think of this self-focused, self-critical frame of mind as *brooding*. Psychologists also call it *rumination*. When we ruminate, we become fruitlessly preoccupied with the fact that we are unhappy and with the causes, meanings, and consequences of our unhappiness. Research has

THE DEFAULT MODE NETWORK

Rumination occurs when a normal daydreaming processes in the brain gets hijacked by negative thinking. What's going on here?

We are creatures of habit, with minds and lives often running on autopilot. This is no accident. There is a network in the brain that has evolved to help us do just that. It's called the *default mode network* (DMN) and involves a group of brain regions including the prefrontal cortex (behind your forehead), parts of the temporal lobe (on the sides), and other inner areas called the *posterior cingulate cortex* and *precuneus*. These work together sending waves of activation to each other and are active when our mind wanders, daydreams, or when we're not focusing on something specific. This helps us be more efficient with our attention. The DMN switches on when we are navigating familiar settings, moving through traffic, or following familiar recipes while still allowing us to plan for the future or listen to a favorite podcast while doing so.

What we tend to forget is that this efficiency comes at a cost. The DMN is always looking for problems to solve—matching situations to habits. This is seen most clearly in brain-scanning studies when the person disengages from an effortful task, such as memorizing words or rotating images. At this point the DMN kicks in. When participants are told that they can "rest and relax," their minds start to wander to stories about themselves, planning, regrets, obligations, and desires. This is how rumination, triggered by the DMN, can feel like productive problem solving, when in fact it is just the mind casting about for a problem that needs fixing, a future plan imagined, or an unfinished goal that needs resolving.

repeatedly shown that if we have tended to react to our sad or depressed moods in these ways in the past, then we are likely to find the same strategy volunteering to "help" again and again when our mood starts to slide. And it will have the same effect: we'll get stuck in the very mood from which we are trying to escape. As a consequence, we are at even higher risk of experiencing repeated bouts of unhappiness.

Why, then, *do* we ruminate? Why, like Carole, do we continue to dwell on thoughts about our unhappiness when it just seems to make things worse? When researchers ask people who ruminate a lot why they do it, a simple answer emerges: they do it because they believe it will help them overcome their unhappiness and depression. They believe that not doing it will make their condition worse and worse.

We ruminate when we feel low because we believe that it will reveal a way to solve our problems. But research shows that rumination does exactly the opposite: our ability to solve problems actually *deteriorates* markedly during rumination. All the evidence seems to point to the stark truth that *rumination is part of the problem, not part of the solution.*

Imagine a car trip during which, every time we check to see how close we are to our destination, we find that the car has instantly moved farther away from it. This is tantamount to what happens in the interior world of emotions and feeling states when we call in the doing mode of mind. That's why we often find ourselves saying things like "I don't know why I feel so depressed; I've got nothing to be depressed about," and then discovering that we feel even more unhappy. We've checked our destination of feeling happy and found ourselves farther away from it. We can't seem to stop reminding ourselves how bad we feel.

SPILT MILK

It was the 1940s, and the Second World War was still raging in Europe. An old dairy farmer in England was talking to a new farmhand who had recently come to help with the cows as part of his rehabilitation after being wounded on the front lines. The farmhand had been learning how to call the cattle back to the barn, lead them into their stalls, give them their food, clean them, milk them, then take the pails full of milk to the cooler and then to the churns. The farmhand was upset because he had spilt some of the milk from the churn and had tried hosing it down with water. As the farmer came around the corner, there was the inexperienced farmhand, gazing in despair at the huge white puddle he had created. "Ah," said the farmer, "I see your problem. Once the water has mixed with the milk, it all looks the same. If you've spilt a pint, it'll look like a gallon. And if you've spilt a gallon, it looks like . . . well, a bit like that lake you're standing in. The trick is just to deal with the milk you've spilt. Let it run off, sweep up what's left into the drain; and then, when it's pretty clear, you can hose it down."

The milk the farmhand had originally spilt was now mixed with the water he'd been trying to clear it up with, and *it all looked the same*. And so it is with our moods. Our best attempts to clear them up can make them worse, *but we don't realize this is what is happening*: it all looks the same and so simply intensifies our desperate attempts to fix things. Nobody waves a flag at us and says, "Wait just a minute; that extra misery you just felt was not part of the mood you were feeling when you started." There is nothing "out there" to remind us that, even with the very best of intentions, we are actually making matters considerably worse for ourselves.

Ironically, as all this is happening, the mood that triggered the whole process in the first place may well have moved on. But we don't notice that it has faded of its own accord. We're too busy trying to get rid of it and creating more misery in our attempts.

∞

Rumination invariably backfires. It merely compounds our misery. It's a heroic attempt to solve a problem that it is just not capable of solving. Another mode of mind altogether is required when it comes to dealing with unhappiness.

∞

THE ALTERNATIVE TO RUMINATION

If Carole had been able to relate differently to the feelings that came over her as she was clearing up her apartment, she might not have gotten lost in the vortex of thinking, thinking, and more thinking. She might have realized that the initial feeling was a passing sadness that often arose when an evening with a friend came to an end. Sadness can arise when friends leave. No further "causes" needed to be unearthed. But we don't *like* to feel sad because it can quickly turn into a sense that we are somehow flawed or incomplete, so we call in the intellect to focus on the mismatch between what "is" and what "should be." Because we can't accept the discomfort of the message, we try to shoot the messenger and end up shooting ourselves in the foot.

There is an alternative strategy for handling the negative moods, memories, and thinking patterns *in the present moment, as they arise.* Evolution has bequeathed us an alternative to critical thinking, and we humans have only just begun to realize its power to transform us. It is called *awareness*.

Mindfulness: The Seeds of Awareness

In a sense we've been familiar with this alternative capacity of ours all along. It's just that the driven-doing mode of mind has eclipsed it. This capacity does not work by critical "problem-solving" thinking but through awareness itself. We call it the *being mode* of mind.

We don't only think *about* things. We also experience them directly through our senses. We are capable of directly sensing and responding to things like the smell of spices, the sound of trucks, and a feel of a cold wind on the skin. And we can be aware of ourselves experiencing. We have *intuitions* about things and feelings. We know things not only with the head, but also with the heart and with the senses. Furthermore, we can be *aware* of ourselves thinking; thinking is not all there is to conscious experience. *The being mode is an entirely different way of knowing from the thinking of doing mode.* Not better, just different. But it gives us a whole other way of living our lives and of relating to our emotions, our stress, our thoughts, and our bodies. And it is a capacity that we all already have. It's just been a bit neglected and underdeveloped.

BEING MODE

Being mode is the antidote to the problems that the driven-doing mode of mind creates.

By cultivating the awareness of being mode we can:

■ Disengage the autopilot in our heads. *Being more aware of ourselves—through the senses, the emotions, and the mind—can help us aim our actions where we really want them to go and make us effective problem solvers.*

■ Get out of our heads and learn to experience the world directly, experientially, without the relentless commentary of our thoughts. *We might just open ourselves up to the limitless possibilities for happiness that life has to offer us.*

■ Start living right here, in each present moment. *When we stop dwelling on the past or worrying about the future, we're open to rich sources of information we've been missing out on—information that can keep us out of the downward spiral and poised for a richer life.*

■ Sidestep the cascade of mental events that draws us down into depression. *When awareness is cultivated, we may be able to recognize at an early stage the times we are most likely to slide into depression and respond to our moods in ways that keep us from being pulled down further.*

■ Stop trying to force life to be a certain way because we're uncomfortable right now. *We'll be able to see that wanting things to be different from how they are right now is where rumination begins.*

■ See our thoughts as mental events that come and go in the mind like clouds across the sky instead of taking them literally. *The idea that we're no good, unlovable, and ineffectual can finally be seen as just that—an idea—and not necessarily as the truth, which just might make it easier to disregard.*

■ Sense when the doing mode is driving us to exhaustion. *We'll be able to see how best to be kind to ourselves, taking a pause to regather and nourish ourselves before choosing what to do next.*

The rest of this book describes in detail how you can cultivate the type of awareness we're talking about. The core skill is mindfulness. It can profoundly change your life.

WHAT IS MINDFULNESS?

Mindfulness is the awareness that emerges through paying attention on purpose, in the present moment, and nonjudgmentally to things as they are. Pay attention to what? you might ask. To anything, but especially to those aspects of life that we most take for granted or ignore. For instance, we might start paying attention to the basic components of experience, like how we feel, what is on our minds, and how we perceive or know anything at all. Mindfulness means paying attention to things as they actually are in any given moment, however they are, rather than as we want them to be. Why does paying attention in this way help? Because it is the exact antithesis to the type of ruminative thinking that makes low moods persist and return.

First, mindfulness is *intentional.* When we are cultivating mindfulness, we can be more aware of present reality and the choices available to us. We can act with awareness. By contrast, rumination is often an automatic reaction to whatever triggers us. It is tantamount to unawareness, being lost in thought.

Second, mindfulness is *experiential, and it focuses directly on present-moment experience.* By contrast, when we ruminate, our minds are preoccupied with thoughts and abstractions that are far away from direct sensory experience. Rumination propels our thoughts into the past or into an imagined future.

Third, mindfulness is *nonjudgmental.* Its virtue is that it allows us to see things as they actually are in the present moment and to allow them to be as they already are. By contrast, judging and evaluating are integral to rumination and the entire doing mode. Judgments of any sort (good or bad, right or wrong) imply that we or the things around us have to measure up in some way to an internal or external standard. The habit of judging ourselves severely disguises itself as an attempt to help us to live better lives and to be better people, but in actuality the habit of judging winds up functioning as an irrational tyrant that can never be satisfied.

By cultivating mindfulness, Carole might become aware of the intricate interconnections between external events, her feelings, her thoughts, and her behaviors, noticing more and more how one can trigger the other and the entire spiral of depression. She might no longer repeatedly feel quite so stuck in a seemingly never-ending depression because she now has new and wiser ways to relate to her experience in the present moment. She might even find a way to be kind to herself in those times that she is feeling most vulnerable, and this in turn might increase her enthusiasm for taking up new interests and making new friends.

As explained in the rest of this book, practicing mindfulness is more than just noticing things around us that we hadn't noticed before. It is learning to become aware of the particular *mode of mind* that gets us stuck when misapplied to ourselves and our emotional life. The following chapters describe practical skills for disengaging from that mode when it is not serv-ing us and shifting to an alternative mode of mind that will not get us stuck. With an increasing ability to sustain mindfulness, we can explore what hap-pens when our emotions are allowed to come and go in awareness with a nonjudgmental attitude and self-compassion.

As you'll see in the next chapter, the practice of mindfulness teaches us to shift into being mode so that we can be more at peace with our emotions. Our emotions are not the enemy, after all, but messages that reconnect us in the most basic and intimate of ways with the adventure and experience of being alive.

Part II

Moment by Moment

Three

Cultivating Mindfulness

A FIRST TASTE

A well-known travel writer was invited to dine at the home of a well-to-do Japanese family. His host had invited a number of guests, letting it be known that he had something of great importance to share. Part of the meal would consist of blowfish, considered a superb delicacy in Japan, in part because these fish are fatally poisonous unless the poison has been removed by a highly skilled chef. To be served such a fish was a great honor.

As guest of honor, the writer received the fish with great anticipation and savored every mouthful. The taste was, indeed, like nothing he had ever eaten. What, asked his host, did he think of the experience? The guest was ecstatic about the exquisite flavor of the fish he had sampled. He did not have to exaggerate, for it was indeed sublime, among the best food he had ever tasted. Only then did his host reveal that the fish he had eaten was a common variety. Another guest, without realizing it, had eaten the blowfish. The "important thing" the writer learned was not how good a rare and expensive delicacy tasted but how amazing ordinary food could be if he paid close attention to each mouthful.

Being Aware

As he ate the ordinary fish, the writer had an extraordinary experience. The experience was brought about by a shift in the way the writer was paying attention and the resulting quality of his awareness. His host had artfully arranged a situation that would ensure this shift. The fundamental lesson of this book is that we can learn how to bring the same quality of attention to any experience and as a result transform the nature of our experience. This type of awareness, known as *mindfulness,* is much more than paying attention more thoroughly. It is paying attention *differently*—changing *how* we pay attention.

If asked, most of us would say we already pay attention—we have to, just to get everything done we need to do. Or, if we have been chronically unhappy, we may also feel that we are already far *too* aware—at least of the pain we feel when we are feeling down. But the kind of attention most of us customarily pay, particularly when depressed, is attention via tunnel vision. Our attention tends to be contracted around a problem to be solved, as discussed in Chapter 2. Everything that the mind tells us is irrelevant to the problem at hand tends to drop out of our field of vision. Through mindfulness we can experience a moment of life for all that it is, instead of letting our thoughts drag us somewhere we weren't going in the first place. Mindfulness can free us from the trap of rumination and endless "driven-doing" that only imprisons us in further unhappiness and depression.

As we said toward the end of the preceding chapter, mindfulness *is the awareness that emerges from paying attention on purpose, in the present moment, and nonjudgmentally to things as they are.* It's a way of shifting from *doing* to *being* so that we take in all the information that an experience offers us before we act. Being mindful means that we suspend judgment for a time, set aside our immediate goals for the future, and take in the present moment as it is rather than as we would like it to be. It means we approach situations with openness, even if we notice that they bring up feelings such as fear. Being mindful means intentionally turning off the autopilot mode in which we operate so much of the time—brooding about the past, for instance, or worrying about the future—and instead tuning in to things as they are in the present with full awareness. It means knowing that our thoughts are passing mental events, not reality itself, and

> Mindfulness is not paying more attention but paying attention differently and more—wisely—with the whole mind and heart, using the full resources of the body and its senses.

that we are more in touch with life as it is when we allow ourselves to experience things through the body and our senses rather than mostly through our unexamined and habitual thoughts.

It may be difficult to believe how limited our usual way of paying attention is. To demonstrate it to yourself, you might like to try the simple exercise on pages 56–57, right now, to get a feel for the vividness of an experience when the mind is intentionally and nonjudgmentally present for its unfolding. If you can, give yourself permission to spend several minutes on this. If you feel you can't do that right now, you might try it a little later, when you do have the time.

If you have time, you might want to do the exercise with another raisin, perhaps even more slowly, staying aware of any tendency to compare the second raisin to the first one rather than experiencing it on its own terms.

What happens when we engage in this simple exercise wholeheartedly? Just as with the blowfish story, it can give rise to a number of important insights. Kam, a participant in a mindfulness class, was struck by the contrast between this exercise and his usual way of eating: "I normally shovel raisins into my mouth when I'm on the run. This was a whole new level."

Gabriela made a similar comment: "I was very aware of what we were doing. I've never tasted a raisin like that before. Actually, I've never

The raisin exercise can show us how much we miss when we cut ourselves off from the rich input of sensory experience.

noticed what a raisin looked like. At first it looked dead and crinkly, but then I noticed how the light struck it in different ways, like a jewel. When I put it in my mouth, it was hard at first to stop myself from instantly chewing it. Then, when I was exploring it with my tongue, I was able to tell which side was which—but there was no taste. Then when eventually I bit down on it—wow, it was absolutely amazing. I'd never tasted anything like it."

So how did this difference arise for Gabriela? "It's not what I normally do," she said. "It's not how I normally eat raisins. I don't put a lot of thought into what I do. I do it automatically. This time I was really focused on what we were doing rather than thinking of other things."

In this simple mindfulness exercise, Kam and Gabriela had a direct sampling of a new way of relating to experience. They had experienced

EATING ONE RAISIN: A FIRST TASTE OF MINDFULNESS

1. *Holding*
- First, take a raisin and hold it in the palm of your hand or between your finger and thumb.
- Focusing on it, imagine that you've just dropped in from Mars and have never seen an object like this before in your life.

2. *Seeing*
- Take time to really see it, gaze at the raisin with care and full attention.
- Let your eyes explore every part of it, examining the highlights where the light shines, the darker hollows, the folds and ridges, and any asymmetries or unique features.

3. *Touching*
- Turn the raisin over between your fingers, exploring its texture, maybe with your eyes closed if that enhances your sense of touch.

4. *Smelling*
- Holding the raisin beneath your nose, with each inhalation drink in any smell, aroma, or fragrance that may arise, noticing as you do this anything interesting that may be happening in your mouth or stomach.

5. *Placing*
- Now slowly bring the raisin up to your lips, noticing how your hand and arm know exactly how and where to position it. Gently place the object in your mouth, without chewing, noticing how it gets into your mouth in the first place. Spend a few moments exploring the sensations of having it in your mouth, exploring it with your tongue.

6. *Tasting*
- When you are ready, prepare to chew the raisin, noticing how and where it needs to be for chewing. Then, very consciously, take one or two bites into it and notice what happens in the aftermath, experiencing any waves of taste that emanate from it as you continue chewing. Without swallowing yet, notice the bare sensations of taste and texture in your mouth and how these may change over time, moment by moment, as well as any changes in the object itself.

7. *Swallowing*
- When you feel ready to swallow the raisin, see if you can first detect the intention to swallow as it comes up, so that even this is experienced consciously before you actually swallow the raisin.

8. *Following*
  ■ Finally, see if you can feel what is left of the raisin moving down into your stomach, and sense how your body as a whole is feeling after completing this exercise in mindful eating.

firsthand the contrast between the habitual doing mind, on the one hand, and, on the other, remaining fully in touch with each moment, in being mode. They were eating and *knowing* that they were eating. They were eating *mindfully*.

Slowing things down and deliberately paying attention to each aspect of our sensory experience can reveal things that we may have never noticed before. The smell of the raisin may be different from what we had imagined. The texture of the raisin on the tongue may be a novel experience. The taste itself is something we may simply have not experienced before in this way, often richer than the taste of twenty raisins shoved mindlessly into the mouth. Being mindful in this way can radically transform the nature of our experience of eating.

If being mindful can so transform our experience of eating, what could it do for the experience of a sad mood? If we can be present for it, with it, and during it, we could bring to that mood a mind that is ready to experience just that moment, *with no presuppositions or assumptions about it whatsoever.* Eventually we may reach the point where every moment of sadness is no longer experienced as a whole life that's going badly—but just as a moment that feels sad. This shift in and of itself will not necessarily make us feel better. But it may very well send us down a different path, one that doesn't lead so inexorably to depression.

Living in the Present Moment

Gabriela and Kam's experiences of eating the raisin illustrate how easily we get catapulted into the mental time travel that keeps us from experiencing the present moment as a moment and makes us stretch it into the past and toward the future.

Gabriela tried the raisin exercise again at home one evening because she'd found it so calming in the class. It had been a frantic day at work. E-mails, video meetings with colleagues in another city, more video conferencing with clients. Eating lunch on the go.

Once home, as her meal was warming in the oven, she took a single raisin from the packet in the cupboard and held it on the palm of her hand. A moment later she was mentally back at her workplace.

I didn't even have time to eat today. Not properly.

Although her intention was to focus on the sight, touch, smell, and taste of the raisin in each moment, her mind actually wasn't there at all. "Instead," she said, "I was back in the chaos of work, replaying it all over and over."

This can't go on. I'm struggling to handle it all.

And these memories of the day—the meetings, then trying to focus, then the interruptions—took her far away from the present moment and awareness of the raisin. This was not something Gabriela chose to do. It was as if her mind just took off and played out its own agenda. She had wondered about phoning a friend to meet up later, but decided she wasn't in the mood.

During such mental time travel, we can easily forget that we are in the present, as we get into thinking about past or future situations. Instead, we become absorbed *within* those ideas of past or future as if we were actually there. We often relive remembered emotions or prelive anticipated ones. Not only do we remove ourselves from the only reality that we can directly experience, the here and now, but we also suffer the agonies of events that are either long past or may never actually happen. No wonder we can end up feeling worse than we started out.

In the being mode of mind we learn we can inhabit the present with a sense of spaciousness; there is no place else we need to be in this very moment and nothing to do other than what is required in *this* moment. Our minds can be dedicated exclusively to awareness of now, allowing us to be fully present with what life offers us in each moment. This does not mean that we are forbidden from thinking about the past or planning for the future; it only means that when we do think about them, we are *aware* that we are doing so.

Viewing Thoughts as Passing Mental Events

The tremendous power of the mind to think *about* things allows us to solve problems mentally before we actually put the solutions into action. It enables us humans to plan and imagine and write novels. The difficulty occurs when we confuse the thoughts *about* things with the things *themselves*. Thoughts involve interpretations and judgments, which are not in themselves facts; they are merely more thoughts.

The fact that we can be thinking about an imaginary chair in our mind and know that it is not the same as the chair in which we are seated in the living room is relatively easy to grasp. But when the mind brings up ideas of things that aren't physically tangible to begin with—such as our worth as individuals—the distinction can be much harder to see. Ideas about our own self-worth are no more real than thoughts about an imaginary chair. If we switch to being mode through mindfulness, we can see this much more clearly. We can learn to observe our thoughts—and our feelings, for that matter—as experiences that come and go in the mind. Just as the sound of a truck on the street outside passes, and the sight of a bird in the sky is momentary, the thoughts that come to us are mental events that naturally arise, stay for a while, and then fade of their own accord.

> Living in this moment and treating our thoughts and emotions as passing messages similar to sounds, sights, smells, tastes, and touch keeps them from drowning out the signals our senses deliver—signals that can keep us off the road to rumination.

This ever-so-simple, yet challenging, shift in the way we relate to thoughts releases us from their control. For when we have thoughts such as "this unhappiness will always be with me" or "I am an unlovable person," we don't have to take them as realities. When we do, we succumb to endlessly struggling with them. The reality is that these ideas are mental events akin to weather patterns that our mind is generating for whatever reason in this particular moment. If we can see and accept them in this way through mindful awareness, we may eventually gain some insight into when and how they appear. But in the meantime, we certainly don't have to treat them as tyrants to be toppled.

Turning Off the Autopilot

After eating the raisin, many people realize how they hardly ever eat mindfully. They become aware of a huge difference between the experience of this single raisin, approached mindfully, and what happens when they normally eat.

Tyra talked of the comparison with her normal experience of eating a raisin.

"I usually eat on the run. I don't mean to, and I even know it's not good for me. But I do it anyway. And if I sit down, then I'm always scrolling on my phone and catching up with messages. Tasting the food I'm eating? No. Hardly ever."

Unawareness pervades our lives. Eating is simply one example. Even though it might engage all our senses, like Tyra we eat with almost no awareness. It's possible to go for weeks on end, eating several times each day, and never even taste our food. We may be eating and talking, eating and reading, or simply eating while thinking of other things. We are fully entangled in the thought stream of the mind and the pressing needs of our daily lives.

> **"Driven-doing" mode can take on a life of its own, especially when we're unhappy. That's why the shift to mindfulness requires intention and takes practice.**

Dieticians have suggested that eating this way is one reason some of us end up overweight: we pay no attention to the body's signals of satiation. Likewise, the patterns of the mind that get us stuck in unhappiness and depression are old, overlearned habits that get pulled up from memory and take control when we're not fully awake and present. We've passed the reins over to the automatic pilot in the mind, creating the conditions in which these subconscious mechanisms can operate freely.

We've all been on autopilot in everyday situations, and we all know that it often takes us where we hadn't planned to go. Let's say we have to deviate from our usual route home to deliver a package. What happens if we drive on autopilot, daydreaming, problem solving, ruminating? Quite likely we'll find we still have the package in the car when we get home. While our mind was elsewhere, the older habit of following the well-worn route home took control. You've probably laughed when you've discovered your grocery bag filled with everything but the item you went out to get, or when you've found yourself driving to your old apartment instead of your new one, or when you reached out to rub a smudge off your little boy's face, forgetting that he's 27.

Awareness keeps the old habits favored by the automatic pilot from having the final say in determining our actions. It even enables us to spot them on the horizon and recognize them for what they are. Ultimately we may even be able to view our ruminative thought patterns with the same detached, self-compassionate amusement with which we view the lapses that make us forget that our kids have grown up, that our best friend has moved, or that we went shopping because we needed milk. In doing mode our mind is so often preoccupied with *thoughts about* what is going on that we may be only vaguely aware of what is actually happening in the present moment. By contrast, being mode is characterized by awareness of the immediate, sensory experience of the present. We are in *direct* contact with life in each moment. This fresh, direct intimacy with our experience is accompanied by an entirely different way of knowing. It is an implicit, intuitive, nonconceptual, direct knowing of what is unfolding as it is unfolding; it is a knowing of what we are doing as we are doing it.

Without this awareness, we're stuck in a groove that gets deeper the longer we tread that path. Our automatic thought patterns take us down the same road over and over, and we respond with the same actions, which bring about the same worsening feelings—every part of the anatomy of depression triggering the others and the whole. Lack of awareness blinds us to other possibilities. In fact, it blinds us to change in general.

Experiencing Things Directly

CHANGE BLINDNESS

Psychologists Daniel Simons and Daniel Levin conducted an experiment on how much people were aware of what was going on around them as they were walking through the campus at Cornell University. An experimenter carrying a campus map asked unsuspecting pedestrians if they could give directions to a nearby building. Halfway through the encounter the psychologists arranged for two people—dressed as construction workers—to walk between the questioner and the pedestrian while carrying a large door. Thus, for a moment, the interviewer was hidden from view behind the door. With practiced skill, at that very moment, a second questioner took the place of the first one. Different person: different clothing, different height, different voice.

How many people being interviewed noticed the change? Only 47 percent in one study and 33 percent in a second study. Clearly, many of these people were not aware of something that was happening right in front of their eyes: the interviewer changing from one person to another. How could this be? When we're interrupted and given the task of responding to a question that requires some problem solving, we instantly lock on to the goal of solving the problem. As we said at the beginning of this chapter, in doing mode the mind selects only that information that is immediately relevant to attaining that goal. Without being conscious of doing it at all, we screen out much of what is available to our senses, even to the extent of not noticing at all the person to whom we are speaking. Psychologists call this *change blindness*.

Doing mode narrows our attention to the issues it is preoccupied with, creating a veil of ideas that ordinarily keeps us out of touch with direct experience. In the experiment just described, it was the narrow focus of attention on only goal-relevant information that led to the questioner's being seen simply as a generic "person asking me for directions" and therefore not really being seen at all. When we eat while still operating in doing mode, most of our attention is absorbed in or colored by thinking related to achieving the goals set by the unfinished business we seem to carry around with us all the time in the background of the mind: daydreaming, planning, problem solving, rehashing, rehearsing. From the narrow goal focus of doing mode, the sights, smells, sensations, and tastes of eating are simply irrelevant and, for that reason, given only scant attention. Most of us are unaware of how much of life we miss as a consequence.

WASHING THE DISHES

Have you noticed how often we mortgage our present moments for some future promise? Take washing the dishes, for instance. When we are in doing mode, we wash the dishes to get them done as soon as possible so that we can move on to the next activity. Chances are, we are also preoccupied with other things, so we don't give washing the dishes our full attention. Perhaps we are hoping to have a moment to ourselves at long last to relax. We may be thinking about having a cup of coffee and how relaxing that will be. If we then come across a dirty pot that we somehow missed (or, even worse, someone *else* finds a dirty pot that we have missed), we might feel irritated because the offending pot has temporarily thwarted our desire to get finished as quickly as possible. Finally we do finish, and maybe we sit down for a moment to have that cup of coffee. But our mind may still be very much locked into doing mode, preoccupied with its various plans and goals. So even while drinking the coffee, it is very likely that we are already thinking of the next task we have to do—return some calls, pay the bills, run some errands, get back to studying—whatever it may be.

For a moment, perhaps out of the blue, we come to our senses and are struck by the empty cup in our hand. *Did I just drink that? I must have. But I can't remember drinking it.* Although we'd been anticipating sitting down to enjoy the drink, we've actually missed it—just as we missed the whole range of sensory experience associated with washing the dishes: the feel of the water, the sight of the bubbles, the sounds of the scrubber against the plate or bowl.

In this way, little by little, moment by moment, life can slip by without our being fully here for it. Always preoccupied with getting somewhere else, we are hardly ever where we actually are and attentive to what is actually unfolding in *this* moment. We imagine we'll be happy only when we get somewhere else, wherever and whenever that may be. Then we'll have "time to relax." So we postpone our happiness, rather than opening to the quality of the experience we're having right now. As a consequence, we may miss the quality of the unfolding moments in our day, just as we missed doing the dishes and drinking the coffee. If we are not careful, we may actually miss most of our life in this way.

Beyond the Usual Goal Focus

Doing mode is all about reaching preset goals, by focusing on the gap between our ideas of where we are now and our ideas of where we want to be. Being mode, by contrast, is not concerned with the gap between how things are and how we want them to be. In principle at least, there is no attachment to achieving *any* goal at all. This nonstriving orientation in itself helps to release us from the narrow goal focus of doing mode. It also has two very important further implications.

First, in being mode there is no need for constant monitoring and evaluation to see whether the state of the world is approximating our idea of the goal state we have set. This is reflected in the *nonjudgmental, accepting quality of the way we pay attention.* In being mode, we discover we can suspend evaluating our experience in terms of how it "should" be or "ought" to be, of whether it is "correct" or "incorrect," of whether it is "good enough" or "not good enough," or of whether we (or others) are "succeeding" or "failing," even whether we are "feeling good" or "feeling bad." Each present moment can be embraced as it is, in its full depth, width, and richness, without a "hidden agenda" constantly judging how far our world falls short of our ideas of how we need it to be. What a relief! But it is very important to be clear that, when we let go of constantly evaluating our experience in this way, we are not left to float, rudderless, without any purpose or aim to our actions. We can still act with intention and direction; compulsive, habitual, unconscious doing is not the only source of motivation available to us. For *we can also take action in being mode. The difference is that we are no longer so narrowly focused on, or attached to, our concepts around our goals.* This means that we may not be quite as upset or as paralyzed when reality does not

---

PEACE

Peace can exist only in the present moment. It is ridiculous to say "Wait until I finish this, then I will be free to live in peace." What is "this"? A diploma, a job, a house, the payment of a debt? If you think that way, peace will never come. There is always another "this" that will follow the present one. If you are not living in peace at this moment, you will never be able to. If you truly want to be at peace, you must be at peace right now. Otherwise, there is only "the hope of peace some day."

—THICH NHAT HANH, *The Sun My Heart*

conform to our expectations or to the goals we have conceptualized, whatever they are. Alternatively, we might in some moments be very, very upset and perhaps even paralyzed. Yet by allowing our awareness to include even those feelings, that very gesture of awareness, as we shall see in the coming chapters, brings with it a new freedom that allows us to *be* with things as they are (including how upset we are feeling) without having to have them be different from how they actually are in this moment.

We have already hinted at a second profound implication of bringing awareness to our persistent, if unconscious, attachment to goals when we shift into being mode: that we may no longer experience in the same way the entire range of unpleasant feelings and emotions that are automatically generated whenever we focus on the discrepancy between how we are feeling and how we want to feel. When we shift from driven-doing mode to being mode, the attendant shift in our awareness can at a stroke cut through the source of much of the additional unhappiness we had been experiencing. This is because, without our knowing it, the driven-doing had been "making extra"—making us unhappy about our unhappiness, fearful of our fear, angry with our anger, or frustrated with the failure of our attempts to think our way out of our suffering. So, shifting into being mode removes one of the primary sources fueling the escalating cycles of dissatisfaction and depression to which we may be vulnerable. No longer so constantly concerned with what is wrong with our experience, we can open to the possibility of feeling a greater sense of harmony and at-oneness with ourselves and the world.

We've been taught that setting goals and working toward them is the way to get where we want to go: to happiness. It may be difficult to believe, then, that *not* clinging to goals, even worthy goals, may be the way out of *un*happiness. But now that we have seen how clinging to the goal of "fixing" what we can so easily think of as our unworthy self falsely draws us into the downward spiral of rumination and depression, perhaps we can see how the nonstriving orientation of mindfulness might help us avoid that trap altogether. It allows us to refrain from judging and condemning our moods and trying to escape from emotions we don't want to be feeling. As a result, we can "pull the plug" on the habit of depressive rumination, and we have a chance to free ourselves from its relentless pull.

Approaching Instead of Avoiding

Nonstriving, as we said, does not mean floating around without a rudder. It means broadening our focus beyond what's needed to reach a particular goal. It also means that instead of triggering fervent efforts to reject the "unacceptable" emotions that pass through us, we meet them with a sense of acceptance. But mindfulness is hardly passive resignation. It is a stance by which we intentionally welcome and turn toward whatever arises—including *inner experiences* that we'd normally fight or try to escape. Approach and avoidance mechanisms are fundamental to all living systems and to the survival of the organism. Approach and avoidance circuitry is wired into specific areas of the brain. Mindfulness embodies approach: interest, openness, curiosity (from the Latin *curare*, "to care for"), goodwill, and compassion. According to mindfulness teacher Christina Feldman:

> The quality of mindfulness is not a neutral or blank presence. True mindfulness is imbued with warmth, compassion, and interest. In the light of this engaged attention, we discover it is impossible to hate or fear anything or anyone we truly understand. The nature of mindfulness is engagement: where there is interest, a natural, unforced attention follows.

The openhearted "approach" attitude of mindfulness provides an antidote to the instinctive avoidance that can fuel rumination. It gives us a new way to relate to ourselves and the world, even in the face of external threats and internal stress. By regaining intentional control of our attention, we can rescue ourselves from becoming stuck in unhappiness and depression.

The raisin exercise offered a hint of what this intentional shift in attention might feel like. What might happen if we extended the approach we took to eating a raisin to the activities of our everyday lives?

Mindfulness of Routine Activities

We want this new way of paying attention to be here for us when we need it so we can respond skillfully to unhappiness and lead fuller, richer, freer lives. How can we do this? We begin by practicing deliberately paying attention to our experience while carrying out previously routine activities in our everyday lives in the same way that we did with the raisin. We might begin by bringing mindfulness to one routine activity per day; try the exercise below.

The idea is to bring a gentle attentiveness to whatever we are doing. As best we can, each time we do whatever it is, we bring a fresh quality of deliberate, moment-to-moment, nonjudgmental awareness to it. The aim is not to be *hyper*attentive or to bring greater strain or self-consciousness to these routine actions. Actually, we may find that bringing mindful awareness to things reduces effort and makes the chosen activity easier.

It is interesting to notice how difficult it can be for us to do this (apparently) simple thing. How do other people experience such an intentional practice of the mundane? Gabriela had practiced becoming more aware of routine activities. She was due to move to a new apartment in a few weeks,

BRINGING AWARENESS TO ROUTINE ACTIVITIES

One way to practice being more mindful is to choose some *routine activity* that we do every day and resolve that each time we do it, we will bring a fresh quality of deliberate and gentle moment-to-moment awareness to the task or activity as best we can. Bringing awareness into these activities of daily living can make it much easier for us to recognize when we are operating in the doing mode, on automatic pilot, and provides us with an instant alternative, namely, an opportunity to enter and dwell in the mode of being. In this way, we are knowing full well what we are doing while we are actually doing it.

Here are some examples of possible activities:

- Washing the dishes
- Loading the dishwasher
- Taking out the garbage
- Brushing your teeth
- Taking a shower
- Doing the laundry
- Driving the car
- Taking the elevator
- Leaving the house
- Browsing social media
- Entering the home or workplace
- Going upstairs or downstairs
- Playing a game on your phone

Please feel free to add your own chosen activities to this list, perhaps choosing one to focus on for one week, then adding a new activity each week.

and she'd organized a get-together for a few friends—a "goodbye party" for the place she'd lived in since moving to the city. She expected the usual rush and chaos. "Yes, it was very busy—and sometimes I thought *Why am I doing this? We could all have gone out for a film and come back here for some pizza and salad.* But then I remembered the raisin—and becoming mindful of anything—any activity at all. Even the small, routine activities. I thought, *I'm doing this anyway. I'm tidying up, getting food out of the fridge, lighting a candle—and it's not taking me any longer to be aware of what I'm doing!*"

What was it that Gabriela was doing differently? It turns out that focusing on just this moment, no matter how apparently trivial the task, had benefits she had not counted on. For one thing, it seemed to "pull the plug" on her tendency to prelive the future. For another, it prevented her mind from getting trapped in the driven-doing mode that she had previously used to avoid imagined catastrophes. This is how she described it:

"Once I realized that it wasn't taking any longer to be mindful, it was a major revelation. I stayed in the present moment. Usually, I'm always thinking ahead, planning and imagining the worst. *Have I got enough food? What about people's diets? What if they can't eat most of this?*"

It was not that Gabriela ever *chose* to worry about what might go wrong. It is just that, when the mind is elsewhere, when we are out of touch with what is happening around us, old mental habits tend to take over and control how we see and what we do from moment to moment. This can color our experience, shaping it below the level of our awareness. We can often feel victimized without realizing that we are actually collaborating in keeping the whole thing going.

As we've seen, slipping back into old patterns of thinking is the primary pathway by which we become stuck in persistent unhappiness. As in eating, washing the dishes, or getting through our to-do list, we easily and mindlessly slip into daydreaming and problem solving. But daydreaming is the first cousin of rumination. So if we've been depressed for long periods in the past, there is a strong chance (particularly when we're feeling unhappy) that our daydreams will slide into well-worn habits of negative thinking. If we don't notice what is actually happening with us right here and right now, our mood may spiral downward without our catching it. The first step to preventing this from happening is to recognize when we are operating on autopilot and to intentionally, as well as we can manage it, step out of it into a more spacious, self-compassionate, and wiser awareness.

Gabriela had discovered this for herself. "The things I was worried about—it's not that they aren't important, but as I started to focus, moment by moment, on what I was actually doing, I realized that I'd already done what I could to prepare for my friends. And anyway, they know me well enough—and they all know to bring their own snacks if they're really worried about eating the wrong thing. So, paying attention with kindness as I got ready—it was so different from how things usually go. So much more enjoyable too."

The Fresh Air of Awareness

For most of us, a typical day involves hurrying from task to task, forgetting that there are other possibilities for us. Even a tiny bit of mindfulness, brought to any moment, can wake us up, thus subverting the momentum of driven-doing for at least one moment—and that's all we need to be concerned about. And here is an important point: *We don't have to stop what we are doing. We simply bring greater moment-to-moment, nonjudging, wise awareness to our unfolding moments.* The solution to our mood problems may not require heroic attempts to change our inner feeling world or the outer world of people, places, and jobs. Rather, it may simply involve a shift in the way we pay attention to all of them.

If you have ever lived in an old house, or know someone who has, you'll know that dry rot is a major concern. If dry rot has got into the wooden fabric of a house, it can be devastating. One of the recurring themes of the surveyors who advise people on how to deal with it is that air circulation is very important. Dry rot spores cannot survive well where there is a fairly constant exposure to fresh air. A surveyor will advise the buyer to install air vents and other devices for keeping the timber well ventilated. The spores are still around and may settle on the wood, but with fresh air around they will not thrive.

> **Even a little bit of mindfulness brought to a single moment can break the chain of events that leads to persistent unhappiness.**

In a similar way, we could say that stress, fatigue, and distressing emotions thrive in the absence of the fresh air of awareness. It is not that, with awareness, they cease to exist, but that awareness puts more space around them, and such spaciousness, like fresh air to the spores, provides an environment in which the self-diminishing and constricting frames of mind no longer thrive. Mindfulness detects them earlier on, sees them more clearly, and notices how they arise and can pass away. It offers us a way of seeing them clearly without having to get caught in them. We don't usually inhabit or even visit this dimension of our own minds, the dimension of awareness itself, in spite of the fact that it is an intimate part of us. Although it is a powerful capacity we all have, we mostly ignore it. In the chapters that follow, we describe more ways to explore this new dimension of our very own minds and hearts.

Four

The Breath

GATEWAY TO AWARENESS

The raisin exercise is simple, but its implications are profound. It shows us that we can transform experience just by changing the way we pay attention. Using all the powers of awareness available to us can break the chain of rumination and may just free us from the cycle of chronic unhappiness. But tapping these powers requires skills that most of us don't have. This chapter and the rest of Part II present mindfulness practices that have proven invaluable for developing our capacity for recognizing when we're being driven by doing mode and for shifting into mindful awareness.

Steadying the Mind

Cultivating the ability to shift modes requires that we learn how we can be fully present right here, right now, whatever the "here and now" presents to us. Sounds good, except for one thing. Much of the time, if things are not going "our way," we don't really want to be in the present moment: we want to be somewhere else, anywhere else. What is more, much of the time it is not so easy to focus our attention on the present moment, even when we attempt it. Our minds tend to be all over the place, leaping chaotically from topic to topic like monkeys leaping from tree to tree through the jungle.

How often have you left one room in your house in search of scissors or your phone and found yourself in another room without any idea what you came in for? How often have you laughed at a joke, thought to share it with a friend, and then, a mere minute or two later, found yourself thinking about a scene from an audiobook you'd been listening to—without any idea how one thought led to the other? The mind seems to have a mind of its own.

Simply waking up to that fact can be an important discovery. But then what do we do? How can we train the mind to be less scattered and more "present," even when it is at the mercy of so many distractions, even in the face of strongly unpleasant circumstances or stress? How do we stabilize and deepen our capacity for paying attention?

We do so by *choosing* where and how we pay attention. And for this strategy to be effective, we will also need to develop a certain degree of *motivation* and a particular kind of *intentionality* so we are not perpetually at the mercy of the mind's ingrained habits of reactivity. But just trying harder isn't the issue, as we will see in the following tale.

THE NOVICE

In a time-honored story set in an ancient Himalayan kingdom, a novice monk was excited at the prospect of meeting his teacher for the first time. He was on fire with questions but sensed that this was not the time to ask them. Instead, he listened carefully to the teacher's instructions. They were brief and to the point. "Get up early tomorrow and climb to a cave you'll find at the top of this mountain. Sit from dawn to dusk and have no thoughts. Use any method you wish to banish thought. When the day is over, come and tell me how it went."

At dawn the next day the novice found the cave, made himself comfortable, and waited for his mind to settle. He thought that if he sat long enough it would become blank. Instead, his mind was crowded with thoughts. Soon he started to worry about failing the task he had been set. He tried to force the thoughts out of his mind, but that just produced more thoughts. He shouted at them to "Go away," but the words echoed noisily in the cave. He jumped up and down, held his breath, shook his head. Nothing seemed to work. He'd never known such a bombardment of thoughts in his life.

At the end of the day he climbed back down, completely dispirited, wondering what his teacher's response would be. Perhaps he'd be dismissed as a failure, unsuitable for further training. But the teacher just burst out laughing at the tale of his mental and physical gymnastics. "Very good!

You have tried really hard and done well. Tomorrow you should go back to the cave. Sit from dawn to dusk having nothing but thoughts. Think of anything you like all day long, but allow no gaps to occur between your thoughts."

The novice was really pleased. This would be easy. He was bound to succeed. After all, "having thoughts" is what had been happening to him all day.

The next day saw him climbing with confidence up to his cave and taking his seat. After a little while he realized that all was not well. His thoughts started to slow down. Occasionally, a pleasant thought would come to mind and he would decide to follow it for a while. But soon it dried up. He tried to think grand thoughts, philosophical speculations, to worry about the state of the universe. Anything. He started to run low on things to think about and even got a little bored. Where had all his thinking gone? Soon the "best" thoughts he could get seemed a little worn, like an old coat that had become threadbare. Then he noticed gaps in his thinking. Oh dear, this was what he had been told to avoid. Another failure.

At the end of the day he felt pretty wretched. He'd failed again. He climbed down the mountain and went to find his teacher, who burst out laughing again. "Congratulations! Wonderful! Now you know how to practice perfectly." He didn't understand why the teacher was so pleased. What on earth had he learned?

The teacher was pleased because the novice was now ready to recognize something of real significance: *You cannot force the mind. And if you try to, you won't like what comes of it.*

There is no need to climb to the top of a mountain to come to this important conclusion on your own. You might like to try this simple experiment right now. Look away from the book for a minute and think of anything you like, *but try not to think of a white bear.* One minute. Make sure that no thought or image of that animal occurs to you.

Has the minute passed? What did you find?

Most people find they can't completely suppress thoughts of white bears. Professor Daniel Wegner and colleagues have shown that when we try to suppress thoughts like this, *what we resist persists:* our attempts to force the mind can rebound in exactly the opposite direction from the one we want. Not only is it difficult to suppress the thought in the first place, but later, if we're *allowed* to think of white bears, the thought of them comes up more often than if we had not been trying to suppress them earlier.

If this is true for neutral thoughts and images such as bears, it's not difficult to imagine what happens when we try to suppress *negative* thoughts, images, and memories of a very personal nature. If we've experienced persistent low mood in the past, we are likely to put a lot of mental effort into keeping negative thinking at bay. Research by Drs. Wenzlaff, Bates, and associates shows that this can work for a little while—but at a huge cost: those who put more effort into keeping negatives out of mind end up being more depressed than those who do not. From such research, many psychologists have confirmed the conclusion long suggested by meditative wisdom: trying to suppress unwanted thoughts is not a very effective way to stabilize and clear our minds.

> To pay attention to the here and now, we need intention, not force.

WHEN INTENTION WORKS BETTER THAN FORCE

How can we possibly steady and calm the mind if force is so ineffective?

All is not lost. Have you ever seen an infant studying her own hand, totally absorbed in exploring this wondrous creation of nature? Her attention can be sustained, apparently effortlessly, for minutes at a time. The mind has a natural mechanism for supporting sustained, vigilant, engaged attention. How do we tap into it?

One way is to give ourselves the gentle challenge of intentionally focusing and refocusing our attention on a single object. Historically, many different objects of attention have been used to gather and steady the mind in this way, from a gently flickering candle flame to a sound such as "om" repeated silently in the mind. Research has revealed that intentionally focusing on just one object in this way can steady the mind by activating the brain networks corresponding to the chosen focus of attention and, at the same time, inhibiting the brain networks corresponding to competing demands for attention, without any need for force. It's as if the brain "lights up" the selected object while also "dimming" the unselected objects.

To take advantage of these basic processes, these natural tendencies of the mind/brain to settle under certain circumstances, we do actually need to make an effort—but it is a certain kind of *gentle effort*. We direct the spotlight of our attention onto our chosen object and then refocus the spotlight on the object over and over again, whenever we notice it has drifted away. This is very different from the goal-oriented striving that tries to steady the mind by forcing certain thoughts into the mind, by pushing other thoughts out, or by erecting a barrier to the entry of unwanted thoughts and feelings. It is a graceful and gentle kind of effort that signals a shift to a mental mode that supports curiosity, interest, and a tendency to explore and investigate. It is tapping into the mind's capacity to approach rather than avoid situations, as we saw in Chapter 3.

Traditionally, this harnessing of the mind's own natural capacities for calm and clarity is nicely captured by the image of a glass of muddy water. As long as we keep stirring the water, it will stay opaque and cloudy. But if we have the patience to simply wait, the mud will eventually settle at the bottom of the glass, leaving clear, pure water above. In the same way, our attempts to steady, calm, or control our mind often merely stir things up and make everything less clear. But we can get out of our own way and stop contributing to the cloudiness of the mind by encouraging it to alight and dwell on a single object of attention for a time. When we intentionally let go of our urge to force things to be a particular way, the mind naturally settles all by itself, leaving us both calmer and clearer.

It's important to select a relatively neutral object as the chosen focus of attention. The object should not be so emotionally charged or intellectually interesting that it disrupts the development of mental steadiness. From ancient times, the breath has served as a convenient object for this purpose. The intention is to attend as best we can to the constantly changing pattern of physical sensations as the breath moves in and out of the body.

The Breath

You might like to try the first mindfulness-of-breathing practice (page 76) now if you're in a position to lie down briefly. If not, try it a little later.

You can also cultivate mindfulness of breathing in a sitting position. Guidance for this practice is given on Track 4 of the audio files at *www.guilford.com/williams3-materials* and on pages 77–78. Some people prefer to

MINDFULNESS OF BREATHING—LYING DOWN

To get in touch with your breath moving in the body right now, lie down on your back and place one hand over your belly (in the region of the navel). You may notice that in this position the abdominal wall rises with the in-breath and falls with the out-breath. See if you can pick up on and feel this movement, first with your hand, then without your hand, just by "putting your mind in your belly." There is no need to control the flow of the breath. Allow it to come and go as it will, sensing as best you can the changing pattern of physical sensations. Rest here in awareness, with the feeling of the breath moving in the body in this way, or however you find the movement of the belly to be with your own breathing.

read it through first, but when you are ready to practice, follow the audio guidance given on Track 4.

It's remarkable and inspiring to think that the practice of focusing on the breath in this way has been followed, somewhere in the world, every day for at least the last 2,500 years. It provides a wonderful foundation for the practice of meditation. Our breathing is with us wherever we go (we can't leave home without it!); no matter what we are doing, feeling, or experiencing, it is always available to help us to reconnect our attention to the present moment. And if, for any reason, the breath is not providing a stable ground for our attention to come back to, we can always choose to return to the part of the body with which we started this meditation (the sensation of touch, contact, and pressure where the body makes contact with the floor and with whatever we're sitting on), and using these sensations as an anchor, moving back to the sensations of the breath if and when we choose.

Learning to focus, refocus, and refocus our attention on the breath offers a wonderful way to learn how we can be fully present right here, right now, in an instant, at any time, with whatever the "here and now" presents to us. Because we can attend to the movements of the breath only in the very moment in which they are arising, attending to the breath holds us in the present and provides a vital anchor line with which we can reconnect to the here and now when we recognize that our mind has traveled far away, to the "there and then."

MINDFULNESS OF BREATHING—SITTING

Track 4 of the audio files at *www.guilford.com/williams3-materials*

Settling

1. Settle into a comfortable sitting position, either on a straight-backed chair or on a soft surface on the floor with your bottom supported by cushions or on a low stool or meditation bench. If you use a chair, sit away from the back of the chair so that your spine is self-supporting. If you sit on the floor, it is helpful if your knees can actually touch the floor, although that may not happen at the beginning; experiment with the height of the cushions or stool until you feel comfortably and firmly supported.

2. Allow the back to adopt an erect, dignified, and comfortable posture. If sitting on a chair, have the feet flat on the floor with legs uncrossed. Gently close your eyes if that feels comfortable. If not, let your gaze fall unfocused on the floor four or five feet in front of you.

Bringing Awareness to the Body

3. Bring your awareness to the level of physical sensations by focusing your attention on the sensations of touch, contact, and pressure in your body where it makes contact with the floor and with whatever you are sitting on. Spend a minute or two exploring these sensations.

Focusing on the Sensations of Breathing

4. Now bring your awareness to the changing patterns of physical sensations in the belly as the breath moves in and out of the body, just as you did lying down.

5. Focus your awareness on the mild sensations of stretching as the abdominal wall gently expands with each in-breath and on the sensations of gentle release as the abdominal wall deflates with each out-breath. As best you can, stay in touch with the changing physical sensations in your abdomen for the full duration of the in-breath and the full duration of the out-breath, perhaps noticing the slight pauses between an in-breath and the following out-breath and between an out-breath and the following in-breath. As an alternative, if you prefer, focus on a place in the body where you find the sensations of the breath most vivid and distinct (such as the nostrils).

6. There is no need to try to control your breathing in any way—simply let your body breathe by itself. As best you can, also bring this attitude of *allowing* to the rest of your experience—there is nothing that needs to be fixed, and no particular state to be achieved. As best you can, simply surrender to your experience as it is without requiring that it be any different.

Working with the Mind When It Wanders

7. Sooner or later (usually sooner), the mind will wander away from the focus on the breath sensations in the belly, getting caught up in thoughts, planning, or daydreams, or just aimlessly drifting about. Whatever comes up, whatever the mind is pulled to or absorbed by, is perfectly okay. This wandering and getting absorbed in things is simply what minds do; it is not a mistake or a failure. When you notice that your awareness is no longer focused on the breath, you might want to actually congratulate yourself because you've already come back enough to know it. You are, once more, aware of your experience. You might like to briefly acknowledge where the mind has been (noting what is on your mind and perhaps making a light mental note: "thinking, thinking" or "planning, planning" or "worrying, worrying"). Then, gently escorting your attention back to the breath sensations in the belly, as you bring awareness to the feeling of *this* in-breath or *this* out-breath, whichever is here as you return.

8. However often you notice that the mind has wandered (and this will quite likely happen over and over and over again), each time take note of where the mind has been, then gently escort your attention back to the breath and simply resume attending to the changing pattern of physical sensations that come with each in-breath and with each out-breath.

9. As best you can, bring a quality of kindness to your awareness, perhaps seeing the repeated wanderings of the mind as opportunities to cultivate greater patience and acceptance within yourself and some compassion toward your experience.

10. Continue with the practice for ten minutes, or longer if you wish, perhaps reminding yourself from time to time that the intention is simply to be aware of your experience moment by moment, as best you can, using the breath as an anchor to gently reconnect with the here and now each time that you notice that the mind has wandered off and is no longer in touch with the abdomen, in touch with this very breath in this very moment.

Maintaining a focus of awareness on the breath as the mind is pulled away by thoughts, feelings, bodily sensations, or external distractions is not easy. But it may seem less of a struggle when we are able to see such fluctuations in the mind as just "what the mind does"—similar to waves on the surface of water. If we see these "mind waves" as both natural and inevitable, then the very going away and coming back of our attention can be seen as the heart of the practice, not a lapse or a deviation or a distraction from it. For such goings and comings can teach us precisely what we need to learn: to *recognize* when we have drifted into the endless strategizing of the driven-doing mode, to *disengage* from it, and to *enter* and dwell in being.

DISCOVERING UNEXPECTED CALM

Vince found that focusing on the breath had a wonderfully calming effect on him the first time he tried it. His mind settled, and he felt calmer than he had in ages. He decided that he would get into the habit of repeating the same practice each lunchtime at work. Each day, he closed his office door and practiced along with the audio guidance. Not only Vince, but the wider world noticed the difference.

"For some time, my boss has been concerned about how stressed I've seemed," he reflected, "saying to me when she sees me, 'You okay? Do you feel all right?' Now, after I have done the practice at lunchtime at work, I feel a lot more relaxed. Yesterday at lunchtime when I opened my door and started work again, the boss popped her head around the door and asked how I was feeling. I said I was feeling okay. 'And I'll tell you this,' she said, 'I can't count the number of people who've come into my office for something and said, 'Vince seems a lot happier in the afternoons.'

"I do interact with a lot of people in my job—people that I need to see about various things. And they've noticed in the afternoons I'm a lot more relaxed and happier. I feel really good about that, because I feel like it when I 'come back' after lunch, but I hadn't realized that it was actually sort of coming out. I knew how I was feeling, but I hadn't realized that everyone else was noticing it as well."

So what was the difference Vince noticed?

"What I notice is that, if I am in a conversation with someone, or a group of people, and I am getting wound up, I can be aware of the breathing, yet carry on the conversation. Like we could be talking just as we are now, and if I get wound up, I sort of bring the breathing into awareness; the breath is here; and it just helps to calm me."

It was not that Vince was *trying* to be a nicer person or to impress everyone at work. It seemed to be a by-product of his making time at lunch to simply sit quietly and focus on his breath. During these periods of formal mindfulness practice, he had experienced something very important, namely, the inherent tendency of the mind to settle once we let go of our attempts to make ourselves feel a particular way. He was finding that this simple practice was then enabling him to deal with situations differently at other times as well and to *respond* intentionally rather than to *react* automatically. He had been learning the difference between allowing the mind to settle and trying to force it to settle.

> Mindfulness meditation allows us to respond creatively to the present moment, freeing us from the knee-jerk reactions that start the cycle of rumination.

The ability of the mind to settle on its own in the way that Vince experienced has been rediscovered countless times by others over the ages. It has two very important implications. First, it gives us a skillful and effective way to let the mind settle into this natural, if unfamiliar, condition. Second, it shows us that a capacity for inner calm and peace is already within each of us and always available. We don't have to do anything special to attain or deserve this particular way of being—all we have to do is stop getting in our own way, to stop stirring up the mind and making it opaque and cloudy. Amazingly, this inner calm and happiness within each one of us doesn't depend on the fortunes and misfortunes that life delivers. It is always here for us to tap into once we have a reliable method for doing so. This can lead to a greater sense of balance and equanimity in the face of the highs and the lows, the pleasures and the pains, that are an inevitable part of life. This is akin to experiencing an innate and genuine capacity for happiness—for yourself and for others—one that doesn't depend entirely on things always going a certain way or on getting the result we think we need. Not that it is easy to remember this innate capacity and connect with it. That takes training of a certain kind.

DEALING WITH THE WANDERING MIND

Meiying felt hopeless. She had tried to meditate by following the breath, and it seemed to make her feel worse because she couldn't control her mind. *My mind is always on the go. It just interrupts me all the time. It's no good.* Meiying ended up in a battle for control of the mind. Such battles show how hard it is to let go of our attachment to the habit-driven doing mode of mind. We are so used to the speed and busyness of our lives that when we deliberately slow things down and give ourselves just one thing to focus on, something in us rebels. And because our mindfulness practice doesn't make the outside world slow down, the busyness of life is bound to crowd in, again and again. So, when we begin a period of formal practice, sooner or later—usually sooner—we discover that our mind echoes the busyness of the world. It is as if the mind has a life of its own. Regardless of our determination to keep it focused on the breath or any other object, it will wander away into various thoughts, often about the future or the past.

This tendency of the mind to wander is perfectly normal. The fact that our thoughts seem to proliferate without end doesn't at all reflect an inability to meditate on our part, even though it can be somewhat demoralizing at first to discover this attribute of our own mind. In fact, this recognition of the ever-changing nature of our own thought stream, and how labile our attention is, marks not the end but the beginning of meditative awareness. All the same, it is very easy to become fidgety in the face of the unrelenting torrent of thoughts and to think that we must be doing something wrong. Like Meiying, we might wind up telling ourselves that nothing useful or interesting seems to be happening; the mind is just wandering uncontrollably, even as we persist in bringing it back over and over again to a sense of the breath moving in the body, or whatever our primary focus of attention may be. "You're no good at this," the mind says to itself.

It's only natural to think that the work of meditation is being interrupted when the mind wanders here, there, and everywhere. Yet it is actually at this point that the meditation practice becomes really interesting and vital. Each moment in which the mind takes off gives us one more opportunity to become more aware of when we are slipping (or have already slipped) out of being mode and back into driven-doing mode. It allows us to become more aware of the thoughts, feelings, and body sensations that carry us away in those moments. Happily, such occasions happen so often that we will have countless opportunities to witness the seething pressure of the driven-doing mind, perhaps perceiving it with greater clarity than ever before, uncomfortable as that may sometimes be. These occasions also provide us, crucially, with valuable opportunities to cultivate the skills of releasing ourselves from driven-doing mode and returning to the more mindful being mode.

This is why the instructions for the mindfulness-of-breathing practices encourage us to congratulate ourselves at first when we notice our awareness is no longer on the breath. In that very moment, it can be helpful to note briefly what is on our mind and name what is going on (for example, "thinking, thinking," or "planning, planning," or "worrying, worrying"). *Whatever the content of the thought or impulse, the task is the same:* to note what is on our mind in this moment and then to gently escort our awareness back to our breathing, renewing our contact with the in-breath or the out-breath, whichever is happening when we come back.

At this point, we may find ourselves judging our experience quite harshly because we may feel so frustrated or thwarted in our efforts. *Why can't I do this better?* we may say to ourselves. In such moments, it helps if we can remember to bring a quality of kindness even to this awareness, seeing that these self-critical and judgmental thoughts and feelings are just more thoughts and feelings, like any others, just old and ingrained weather patterns in the mind and of no particular import or significance. Nor are they accurate. But their presence can be seen as providing multiple opportunities and reminders for us to bring patience, gentle acceptance, and openness to our experience. And why not do so, since our experience is already as it is? Being harsh with ourselves because we don't like how it is, is adding something extra and is unnecessary. Our judging, if not held in awareness in this way, may be exactly what is preventing us from seeing clearly in this moment and from being okay with things as they are.

For this reason, in our recent work, we have been exploring *taking a deliberate pause* when we find the mind has wandered, noting where the mind has gone, and there and then cultivating a sense of appreciation for the mind. We may even thank the mind for the fact that it's trying to do its job as best it can. For whatever the mind brings us when it wanders off, the underlying processes are ones that we need in much of our lives—remembering, planning ahead, knowing where we are now and what we need to be doing next. The mind is also very sensitive to incompleteness and will tend to bring us memories of tasks that have not yet been finished—sometimes from weeks, months, and even years ago. This can bring up a great deal of unpleasant thoughts, but even here, the underlying processes of the mind are trying to help, doing what they're trained to do—exercising skills that we couldn't do without. So even if we find it difficult to be grateful to the mind at these points, we may still bring a little understanding to it, and in that understanding may come a glimmer of kindness and a different perspective on what's happening.

TURNING DISCOVERY INTO EXPECTATIONS

Just like anything else, meditation can all too easily be taken on in doing mode. Perhaps having experienced the turbulence in the mind abating a bit on its own on a few occasions, we may find ourselves expecting it to happen every time we sit down to meditate. If a time comes when we don't feel so settled, we might feel disappointed and frustrated. At some level we may know that putting aside our expectations would be much more effective, yet we can't help asking ourselves, *If we experienced calmness last time, why not now?* Unwittingly, we have slipped into becoming goal-oriented in the meditation practice. Then we may wind up feeling even more strongly that we aren't making any headway with all this meditation practice, that we are right back at square one.

"Sometimes I can get really irritated with it," said Tyra. "I do my meditation when I come home from work. I usually feel very positive about the whole thing, but sometimes I can get so restless, you know, I can get really irritated."

What is actually going on with Tyra? Well, first, there is the restlessness itself. This is a bundle of body sensations accompanied by an internal "feeling." But then along comes something else, something extra: irritation. How had she handled this when it came up? "I tried just to let it be and do what we're doing—just coming back to the breath. Part of it was good, you know. But then I started feeling restless and irritated again."

Irritation is closely associated with frustration, and frustration arises when an expectation or a goal is thwarted. Where had Tyra's goal come from?

"Parts of it just felt wonderful," she said of the practice. "I could get it in snatches, as if I was really here, and then at other times I could feel the irritation."

Without realizing it, Tyra had set a goal of "feeling good" while doing the practice. It's very common to have a feeling that we've "got it" in those moments when we feel calm, that "this" must be what I am really supposed to be feeling, only to feel at other moments like we've "lost it," maybe even in the very next moment. This too is a very common experience in meditation practice, and not a problem at all, especially if we can be aware of it and smile inwardly at the unending antics of our own doing mind. But once we have felt a sense of peace, even for the briefest of moments during a session of practice, the doing mind's habitual tendency to look for goals naturally kicks in and generates the expectation or hope that we will have the same experience in the next moment or the next time we do the practice. And if that experience doesn't repeat itself according to our expectations, how easily we can feel disappointment and irritation—sometimes subtle, other times more obvious. Even if we recognize the expectation and the irritation, we can still easily feel critical of ourselves for getting irritated. The gyrations of the judging mind are truly endless, and so off-base from simply accepting things as they are. We may even wind up thinking that experienced meditators never feel irritated, as we generate endless fantasies and idealizations about meditation.

> Consciously acknowledging the mind wandering reminds us that we've already returned our attention to the present moment and makes it easier to let go of the tendency to judge ourselves harshly for not "doing it right."

So if irritation arises in any moment, it may be helpful not to take the route of judgment and fantasy, but rather simply to note it as "irritation," labeling it as a way of acknowledging it for what it is. Then we can gently redirect our attention back to the breath.

Our expectations of "what we *ought* to be feeling" will habitually and automatically rear their old, familiar heads and, on occasion, in our unawareness, cause us to feel frustrated. The challenge in such moments is simply to note the "coulda, shoulda, woulda, oughta" thoughts with friendly interest as old acquaintances. We can simply recognize them as "thinking" or "judging" or "berating" and return our attention to the breath, or whatever part of the body we had chosen as an anchor.

Over time these goal-driven mind states will become more familiar and less of an enemy or an obstacle. Although the sense of struggle can come back with exasperating regularity, gradually our recognition of such antics becomes more of a friendly reminder of just how much power the driven-doing mode exerts over our lives, and even our thoughts and feelings and motivations. Rather than a reason to despair, however, such goal-driven and judgmental mind states can be treated as cues, reminding us of how easy it is to get caught in difficult emotions around "getting somewhere" or "making progress." This is how we eventually learn to view our thoughts and feelings as just thoughts and feelings, as described in Chapter 2—and come to see that they are usually neither particularly accurate nor helpful.

ACCEPTING MIND WANDERING AND STARTING OVER

When practicing mindfulness, if we slip back into the doing mindset, thinking that the meditation is "not working" or that we are "doing it wrong," it can be very helpful to remind ourselves that cultivating mindfulness of breathing, or any other object of attention, is fundamentally a practice of beginning again, and again, and again each time we are caught up and carried away by the wanderings of the mind.

"I can see that my mind wanders away," said Vince. "It can last some time before I realize what is happening. What I used to do is get angry and frustrated about it. Now I tend to notice that the mind drifts around quite a bit.

"So I let the thoughts drift past, and if I can bring myself back even a little, the thoughts don't bother me so much. They used to be really intense, whereas now they're sort of just floating around."

Vince has learned to notice the drifting and bring his attention back to the body and breath without giving himself a hard time about it. He has stopped getting so frustrated by the fact that his attention tends to get hijacked by his various thoughts. Not that it doesn't continue to happen. But learning to witness this whole process without reacting to it so

If you find yourself feeling frustrated by the mind's wanderings . . .

remind yourself
that mind-wandering is
simply the doing mode at work;
that the moment of recognizing it
is itself a moment of mindfulness.

If you find yourself feeling "I should be better at this by now" . . .

remind yourself
to note the "shoulda, coulda, woulda, oughta" thoughts—
the judging mind—
and return to the breath.

If you find that you are trying to control the breath . . .

remind yourself
to let it breathe itself.

automatically has allowed him to refocus on the sensations of breathing much more reliably than when he is caught up in being self-judgmental.

Much of the struggle with the practice comes just at the moment when we are already back in the present moment and realize that the mind has been absorbed in wandering. But this moment is also a major opportunity for learning. Through repeated practice we see over and over again that each in-breath is a new beginning and each out-breath a fresh let-

> Beginning again does not mean we have made an error. It is the heart of the practice, not a deviation from it.

ting go. We begin to see that the shift from one mode of mind to another can be virtually instantaneous. In this way the practice is always giving us the chance to begin again, in this moment, with this breath. If our mind wanders 100 times during a period of formal practice, then we simply, and good-naturedly, bring it back 100 times. This is what Vince was reporting about his experience.

Eventually we may come to see what this practice is actually asking of us: to recognize and accept that our mind does indeed have a life of its own and that it will inevitably wander away from whatever object of attention we set for ourselves—in this case, the breath. And we may come to see that we can gently escort our attention back to the breath every time this happens. Ultimately, we come to see that we can cradle all of it in awareness with a light and gentle touch, including the wandering of the mind, with all its obsessions and its struggles. Just that. And *that* is a lot, perhaps everything. We may come to realize that our moments of greatest struggle can be our moments of greatest learning. In the moment of beginning again, even when we've been struggling, we may experience a fleeting sense of joy, a feeling perhaps of coming home or of recognizing an old friend. Such experiences can awaken our curiosity and our sense of adventure and keep us practicing when part of us feels like giving up.

LETTING BE, ALLOWING: GIVING UP CONTROL

Suzanne found it hard to focus on the breath without trying to control it: "I find that I'm trying to control my breath to make it slower. I'm thinking all the time about whether it is right. It doesn't feel to me like natural breathing."

Trying to control the breathing is not an uncommon experience in the early stages of meditation practice. But again, the body knows how to breathe just fine on its own. In fact the breath does what it has to do perfectly . . . *until* the thinking, doubting, striving mind gets involved. Then we find it terribly difficult to ease up on ourselves and let go of our expectations of how things "should be." We find it difficult to trust that, left to itself, the breath will sort itself out.

Eventually Suzanne realized that she did not have to try to slow down her breathing, that she did not have to do anything different—that, in fact, she didn't have to *do* anything at all. She began to focus on the sensations that go along with breathing, instead of trying to control the breath to make something happen.

"I quite enjoy it now," she said. "I used to try to consciously control it all: to control this and control that or control the breathing. Then I found in the end it became easier to let the breathing just happen and to bring myself back when it wandered. If you are not getting wound up in some thought pattern, it's easier."

There is no particular state we need to achieve when practicing mindfulness of breathing—the idea is simply to allow the experience of each moment to be just as it is without requiring that it be any other way. In other words, to be aware and to settle into and dwell in that awareness.

TAKING IT BREATH BY BREATH: ONLY THIS MOMENT

Focusing on the sensations of breathing as one breath follows another teaches us how to take one thing at a time and be in one moment at a time. In everyday life we encounter many situations where we tend to anticipate the future. It is like facing a pile of logs that has to be moved. If we look at the whole pile, our heart sinks, our energy may fail, and doing something else (anything else!) will suddenly seem more attractive than it had before. But we also know that if we are able to focus on the one log we've got to move in this moment, and give our full attention to that, and then take on the next one, all of a sudden the chore becomes doable. The point is not simply to fool ourselves into pretending the pile is not large, but to explore the possibility that we can enter a different mode of mind, a mode in which we attend to the quality of the present moment, rather than anticipating how exhausted we may feel at the end.

The pile-of-logs effect applies to much of our lives. We often exhaust ourselves by focusing on all the things we have to do, not just for this day, but for the weeks or the months ahead. We carry a burden that doesn't need to be carried. When we deliberately tune in to just this moment, to what is before us right now, we allow the energy to come through to complete just this moment's task.

Mindful Walking

Nearly all the practices described in this book include a deliberate focusing of attention in the present moment, on one aspect of our experience or another. In that way these practices help steady the mind as we cultivate mindful awareness. Indeed, some steadiness is essential whenever we wish to relate to our experience with greater clarity and awareness. But there may be times when our minds are too agitated or driven to focus effectively on the breath while the body is sitting or lying still. At such times it can be invaluable to turn to another equally familiar aspect of everyday experience: the sensations in the body as we walk. Since ancient times, mindful walking has been used in tandem with mindful breathing. It is also a wonderful meditation practice in its own right.

You may already be familiar with how a meditation that involves moving, like mindful walking, can shift us from one mental mode to another. Tai chi, chi gung, and hatha yoga are all moving meditations. Perhaps for you walking the dog or going out for a run has been a good way to "clear your head" when you're stuck in a vicious mental circle while trying to come up with a creative idea. Or perhaps you can recall how dancing at a weekend party had you feeling fully alive in that moment, relieved of the cumulative burden of the past week's problems. Or maybe you just know that doing something physical when you're upset helps you "let off steam" and avoid being sucked into endless brooding. All of these physical activities are in themselves potential mindfulness practices, when they are engaged in with awareness and an intentional shift in attention. Walking meditation is a powerful way to cultivate mindfulness while moving, as we shall see in the practice described on pages 90–92 and in the audio guidance on Track 8 at *www.guilford.com/williams3-materials*.

There are many different ways to practice mindful walking and many different places where we can allow our attention to settle and return to when it goes off. One is to focus attention on the sensations associated with the feet moving during walking and especially with the moments of contact with the floor or ground. You might want to take some time to practice this now, after reading the instructions that follow. Or you might want to try it at some other time.

LEARNING FROM WALKING

Walking practice turns out to be especially useful when we feel agitated and unable to settle or when we just can't sit still any longer. The physical sensations of walking can also help us feel more grounded emotionally in difficult times than we might feel in the sitting meditation practice. Mindful walking has been described as "meditation in motion." The invitation is to be, and be mindful, with every step, to walk for its own sake. That is one reason for walking up and down a few paces on the same path without any

MINDFUL WALKING

Track 8 of the audio files at *www.guilford.com/williams3-materials*

Preparation

1. Find a place (indoors or outdoors) where you can walk back and forth in a lane, in a location that is protected enough so that you will not be preoccupied by a feeling that other people are watching you do something they (and even you at first) may perceive as strange.

2. Stand at one end of your walking lane, with your feet parallel to each other, body-width apart, and your knees "unlocked" so they can flex gently. Allow your arms to hang loosely by your sides or hold your hands loosely together in front of your body or behind it. Direct your gaze, softly, straight ahead.

3. Bring the focus of your awareness to the bottoms of your feet, getting a direct sense of the physical sensations of the contact of the feet with the ground and of the weight of your body transmitted through your legs and feet to the ground.

Beginning to Move

4. Allow the left heel to rise slowly from the ground, noticing the sensations in the calf muscles as you do so, and continue, allowing the whole of the left foot to lift gently as the weight is shifted entirely to the right leg. Bring awareness to the sensations in the left foot and leg as you carefully move it forward and allow the left heel to come in contact with the ground. A small, natural step is best. Allow the rest of the left foot to make contact with the ground, experiencing the weight of the body shifting forward onto the left leg and foot as the right heel comes off the ground.

5. With the weight fully transferred to the left leg, allow the rest of the right foot to lift and move it slowly forward, aware of the changing patterns of sensations in the foot and leg as you do so. Focus your attention on the right heel as it makes contact with the ground. Be aware of the weight now shifting forward onto the whole of the right foot as it is placed gently on the ground, and of the rising of the left heel again.

Walking

6. In this way, slowly move from one end of the walking lane to the other, aware in particular of the sensations in the bottom of the foot and the heel as they make contact with the ground and of the sensations in the muscles as each leg swings forward. You can also expand your awareness whenever you care to, if it seems appropriate, to include a sense of what the breath is doing in the various phases of the walking, when it is coming in and when it is going out, as well as the sensations of breathing. Your awareness can also include a sense of the body as a whole walking and breathing, as well as of the changing sensations in the feet and legs with each step.

7. When you come to the end of the lane, stop for a moment or two and just be aware of standing; then turn slowly around, aware of and appreciating the complex pattern of movements through which the body changes direction, then mindfully continue walking. You might also notice from time to time what the eyes are drinking in as your position changes and you receive whatever the view is that is in front of you.

8. Walk back and forth in this way, sustaining awareness as best you can of the full range of your experience of walking, moment by moment, including the sensations in the feet and legs, and of the contact of the feet with the ground. Keep your gaze directed softly ahead.

When Your Mind Wanders

9. When you notice that the mind has wandered away from awareness of the experience of walking, gently escort the focus of attention back to whatever aspect of the walking you are attending to as your object of attention, using it as the anchor to bring your mind back to the body and to the walking. If the mind is very agitated, it is helpful to stop for a moment and just stand here, with feet body-width apart, in touch with the breath and the body as a whole standing, until both mind and body restabilize themselves. Then resume the mindful walking.

10. Continue to walk for ten to fifteen minutes, or longer if you wish.

11. To begin with, walk at a pace that is slower than usual, to give yourself a better chance to be fully aware of the sensations of walking. Once you feel comfortable with walking slowly with awareness, you can experiment with walking at faster speeds up to and beyond normal walking speed. If you are feeling particularly agitated, it may be helpful to begin walking fast, with awareness, and to slow down naturally as you settle.

12. Remember to take small steps in the walking. And you don't need to look at your feet. They know where they are. You can *feel* them.

Ending

13. When you are ready, bringing this period of walking to an end. As often as you can, bring the same kind of awareness that you are cultivating in walking meditation to your normal, everyday experiences of walking. Of course, if you are a runner, you can always bring a similar quality of attention to the step-by-step, moment-to-moment, breath-by-breath experience of running you have cultivated in the mindful walking.

destination. The absence of a destination or goal builds on the same theme as when we begin over and over again with each in-breath and each out-breath: it reminds us that there are alternatives to modes of mind that are centered on doing, in which we always have to be getting somewhere. The simple walking back and forth along the same path embodies the theme of "nowhere to go, nothing to do, nothing to attain." It is simply being here fully in this moment, with this step.

"I like the walking meditation," explained Suzanne, "because I can be conscious of it when I travel to and from work—walking between the office and the parking. I often find I'm in a rush and getting a bit stressed. Sometimes now I'll be aware of it, and I'll walk more slowly and, you know, breathe with the steps. So by the time I actually get to wherever I'm going, I'm calm."

Sometimes she found it helped to sit in the car for a moment or two and just be aware of her breathing before getting out: "You end up with your mind sort of whizzing round, and then your activity goes up and, you know, your body is whizzing around. If I slow down, everything else slows down and I become more aware of what's going on. It doesn't matter if I am a few seconds late. When you become aware of time, I think, one minute can be a very, very long time, when you want it to be."

Of course, once Suzanne had shifted into walking with awareness, she could have walked quickly with full awareness. But slowing the body did help to settle things for her. Suzanne's experience shows how we may use any small moments to be mindful. For her, mindful walking helped to transfer what she was learning from her quieter, more regular mindfulness practice at home to the hurly-burly of everyday life.

From Unawareness to Awareness

The novice we met in the story earlier in this chapter had tried to control his mind, first by emptying it of thoughts, then by filling it with thoughts. Focusing on either goal and judging how close he was getting to achieving it meant he had no peace. We practice sitting with the breath or walking mindfully to help us become more aware, not as a strategy to clear the mind of thought or anything else. Clarity and steadiness of the mind may follow as by-products of such awareness and from allowing things to be as they are, but if we take momentary calmness as a sign of how much progress we are making and momentary restlessness as a sign of lack of progress, we are merely sowing the seeds of further frustration and despair, for we are letting the doing mind compare our "achievement" with some desired "outcome." As long as we are trying to get rid of unpleasant thoughts or feelings or trying to achieve peace of mind, we will continue to be frustrated.

The intention in mindfulness practice is not to forcibly control the mind but to perceive clearly its healthy and harmful patterns. It is to approach our minds and bodies with a sense of curiosity, openness, and acceptance so that we may see what is here to be discovered, and be with it without so much struggling. In this way, little by little, we begin to release ourselves from the grip of our old habits of mind. We begin to know directly what we are doing as we are doing it. We are beginning a graceful transition from unawareness to awareness.

Five

A Different Way of Knowing

SIDESTEPPING THE RUMINATING MIND

"That really tickles me."

"My heart soared."

"I just feel sick about what happened yesterday."

"My heart sank."

"I have butterflies in my stomach."

"My heart stopped."

We use metaphors like these to convey our emotional states for good reason. The body and its infinite sensations are the repository of and the messengers for emotion. Joy, pleasure, or amusement can actually feel something like a tickle. Of course, the heart doesn't move around in the body when we feel "uplifted" or "beaten down," but some real physical sensations occur that are captured by those descriptions. Nor does the heart stop when we're shocked or frightened, but the emotional signal is so strong that we may momentarily feel like it has.

The point is that the body has a lot to tell us about how we are feeling, not just at peak moments but all the time. Yet we often don't hear its messages with any degree of wisdom, because we are too busy reacting to them in ways that immediately trigger a cascade of thoughts and judgments. The challenge here is whether we can, in the being mode, actually open to, know, and befriend the very sensations and feelings we are experiencing in the body, whatever they may be, and accept them with a new receptivity because they are actually part of the sensory landscape of our own body in this moment. If we can listen with this kind of openness, we will discover powerful new ways to *be with* what we are experiencing in any moment, whether it is pleasant, unpleasant, or neutral.

"I feel the weight of the world on my shoulders," we sometimes say. We may be more familiar with that sensation than many others—and certainly more often than we'd like. This is how many of us feel when depressed or unhappy—as if a huge burden has been placed on the body, making every normal action an effort. In Chapter 1 we talked about the importance of the body in the anatomy of depression. Through the raisin exercise and mindful walking, perhaps you've had a chance to see how out of touch we can be with our direct sensory experience, including the body's various messages. A rich and varied landscape is available to us when we open to these aspects of the present moment, grounded in the body itself, and not simply carried away by the mind's reactions in thought and emotion.

As we discussed earlier, physical sensations, thoughts, feelings, and behavior all work together to create a state of depression. Let's focus for a moment on the way that sensations in the body can trigger negative thinking. Consider how you might feel upon waking up when you've been feeling down for a stretch of time. Perhaps the first thing you notice is how heavy and achy your body is. Maybe you don't even feel rested after a night's sleep. Your energy level is so low that you actually feel more tired than when you went to bed the night before. Maybe this has been happening to you a lot lately.

In addition to these sensory aspects of your experience, thoughts like *I don't think I'm going to get anything done today* or *Another wasted day* may waft through your mind. Perhaps such thoughts lead you to feel frustrated and sad, disappointed with yourself. Eventually you try to get out of bed but feel so heavy and tired that you drop back from the very effort. Maybe you try to put the thoughts of how listless you feel out of your mind. You certainly don't want to feel like this. You're fed up with these daily battles with lack of energy. *I've got to get up and get going; this is doing me no good at all,* you might hear yourself say. When you finally do get up, the listless feeling may pass as you busy yourself with the day's activities. But these morning struggles seem to be an increasing burden.

In Chapter 1 we talked about how physical sensations, thoughts, feelings, and behavior can coalesce in the downward spiral of depression. If we look more closely at what is happening in the preceding scenario, we can see that if the morning starts with sensations of physical sluggishness, then thoughts *about* this sluggishness may surface along with emotional reactions. The effects of these emotions in the body only strengthen the sense of physical heaviness. This scenario illustrates how easily we can get trapped in a cycle in which our thoughts about our body sensations can drag us down into depression.

But what if we could open ourselves to the full panoply of direct sensory experience instead of simply getting carried away by the mind's reactions in thought and emotion? We've seen how the messages from our senses seem to acquire new dimensions when we bring mindfulness to them in the present moment—how eating a raisin can become a novel sensory, even sensual, experience or how walking reveals itself to be a mechanical, tactile, and kinesthetic miracle. If we can come to know sensations and feelings directly, befriending the sensory landscape of our own body, we will have a powerful new way to experience and be in wiser relationship to *every* moment, including the moment when we wake up, whether our experience of that moment is pleasant, unpleasant, or neutral. In this chapter we delve more deeply into mindfulness of body sensations, focusing in particular on the ways in which mindfulness offers us new possibilities for knowing the body and for avoiding the traps by which our usual habits of thinking about the body ensnare us.

Sensation through Direct Experience . . .
Instead of Thinking

The machinery that sets the cycle of unhappiness in motion may operate so smoothly that we don't even detect its workings, but that does not mean that it is an unstoppable juggernaut. Every link that keeps the machine going—body–thoughts, thoughts–feelings, feelings–body, and so forth—is an opportunity to redirect the sequence. The cycle can be broken simply by bringing mindful awareness to its links and, in particular, to the body. This may be hard to believe. Truthfully, the only way to confirm it is through your own experience. If right now you're thinking that you are *already* aware of your fatigue—too aware of it, in fact—it may be helpful to recall the theme sounded in Chapters 2 and 3, namely, that mindfulness is not just about paying *more* attention, but rather about cultivating a *different*, wiser kind of attention.

As we have seen, in doing mode we see the world only indirectly, through the veil of our thinking and labeling. If we think about our bodies in the usual way (from the perspective of our heads), then as soon as we feel listless on awaking, our mind fills with ideas *about* the body, what is going on in our lives, everything. This way of paying attention will just make things worse. If, instead, we begin to focus on the body from the perspective of being mode, we open to a direct sensing of the body itself. Moment by moment, we can become aware of body sensations but now in a new way, *a way that does not keep us so stuck obsessing in our thoughts about how we are feeling in the body.* This can help our feelings of sluggishness to dissipate or dissolve, like a fog lifting. We don't have to make them go away. Sooner or later, they will inevitably fade on their own because we are no longer feeding them with incessant negative thinking, without even realizing it. In the process, we shift from feeling powerless in their presence to having viable ways to be in a different relationship to them or anything else that arises—a relationship that is kinder, wiser, and sees what's happening from a wider perspective.

> When the mind instinctively responds to physical sensations with ideas *about* the body, the stage is set for rumination to begin. Mindfulness provides us with another way to know our bodies, one that will not get us stuck.

Mindfulness involves settling into awareness itself, which is as different from thoughts and feelings as the sky is different from the clouds, birds, and weather patterns that pass through it. It is a bigger container, in which all the other events of mind and body unfold. It is a different way of knowing, a different way of being. It is a capacity that we all already have, one that is innate to being human. And we can learn to trust it. We can practice resting in awareness more, in this way of knowing and being. We might even find that this awareness itself offers a certain kind of shelter or refuge from the stress and strain of life, freeing us from the habitual and vicious cycles of the doing mode and the clouds of depression that hang over us.

As we've said, doing mode and its thinking patterns tend to obscure the experiential quality of being mode. This has always been the case. But the extraordinary developments in digital technology that have occurred—even since the first edition of this book was published (the same year as the iPhone)—have brought about a revolution in how we communicate and a revolution in how we use our "downtime." The advantages of greater communication for many have brought major benefits, yet moving further away from physical experience can be challenging, stressful, and reduce well-being in subtle ways.

Mindfulness training involves extensive practice in getting in touch, moment by moment, with the direct experience of life unfolding, without rejecting or clinging to whatever might be distracting us—technological or not. The body is a great place to start cultivating this new way of being. The very physicality of raw bodily sensations provides an ideal base from which to develop a new, more direct, experiential, sensory way of knowing.

Somewhat amazingly, we can bring mindfulness to our experience of the body in any moment, under any circumstances. We can even begin as we sit right here, right now, through the following simple experiment.

Choose a part of the body and think about it for a moment. Let's say we focus on the hands, thinking about them without actually looking at them. Usually, when we think about our hands, the picture we have of them in our minds is as we normally see them, from the perspective of our eyes in our head. It's as though we are the observer up in the head. We know where the hands are and what they look like, but we're a bit separated from them. We may find ourselves having lots of thoughts about our hands. We may like or dislike the shape of our hands; we may find ourselves thinking about how our hands or fingernails compare with those of our friends or how they are aging. But what if we approach our hands in a different way, described on page 99?

From this little exercise, did you notice any difference between thinking *about* your hands and sensing them *directly*? One feature of direct sensing is that the feelings coming from your hands may not be "hand-shaped"—we may simply experience our hands as patterns of different sensations: pressure, warmth or coldness, tingling or numbness.

This distinction between *thinking about* the body and *directly experiencing* the sensations in the body is critically important. Often we see the body as if from a lofty citadel in the head. We look down on the body (physically and metaphorically) and think "Oh, yes, there's a bit of a pain there, a bit of an itch there—I must do something about it." But there is a different

MINDFUL AWARENESS OF THE HANDS

After thinking *about* the hands, now bring your attention right *into* your hands, whatever position they are in at this moment, without looking at them. Allow your awareness to fill your hands from inside to outside, from the bones right out to the skin itself and the fingernails. Open in awareness to any and all sensations in the fingertips, in the fingers, sensing the air between and around the fingers, feeling how it feels on the backs of the hands and in the palms, the thumbs, and the wrists. Also, open to the sense of touch wherever the hands make contact with an object, such as with your knees, if your hands are resting on them, or with the chair or cushion. Note the tactile elements and the temperature, any sense of hardness or softness, of coolness or warmth—whatever is present.

Now move your hands to the chair on which you are sitting, gently touching the side of the chair with the fingertips, very lightly, maintaining awareness of the sensations in the fingers. Now, gripping the sides of the chair, pay attention to the physical sensations in the body where you're gripping. Bring awareness right down into the fingers and hands, directly sensing the contact with the chair, the pressure in the fingers where they are gripping it, exploring with awareness the actual contact between the fingers and the chair. Feel the tightness in the muscles, perhaps a sense of coolness or tingling and a flux of other sensations. And now just ease off and, keeping the awareness in the hands, see if there is any change in the sensations as you move the hands back to your lap or thighs. Then for the last few moments, continue to allow your attention to rest in your hands to feel what's going on in your hands right now.

possibility. We can learn *to bring the mind right into the body* and inhabit the whole of it with awareness.

WHAT CAN WE LEARN FROM DIRECT BODILY EXPERIENCE?

Let's look at Nancy's experience with the preceding experiment. In the first part of the exercise, Nancy was able to get a picture of what her hands looked like quite easily—she had been thinking a lot lately about how worn out she looked, and she had noticed that her hands were beginning to look tired and old. Thinking about her hands brought back memories: she remembered her mother's hands, so strong and powerful when Nancy was a child and so old and weak when, many years later, Nancy was caring for her mother. That was twenty years ago. Now it was Nancy's turn to have the old hands, to feel that life was slipping by. Thinking and memory, so much a part of the doing mode's way of knowing, had already taken Nancy quite a distance away from the immediacy of her present experience.

In the second part of the experiment, Nancy found herself directly tuning in to the sensations in her hands. She noticed some tingling in her fingers, and although at first she started to wonder whether this might mean circulation problems, she was able to come back to simply focusing on the sensations. She noticed that the tingling had faded, and her hands now felt warm—but the warmth came and went as she focused her attention on the sensations. When she touched the chair, she had a sense of the coolness of the metal and a slight numbness as she gripped it. She became quite absorbed in noticing the way the sensations from her hand did not feel handshaped—this was a new experience for her. At the end of the exercise, she realized that her mind had been quite focused and that it had not wandered so much. Her focus on directly sensing the body seemed to have temporarily weakened the chatter of her mind; the direct experiential knowing of the being mode meant that she was able to stay closer to her immediate, bare experience and was less likely to get carried away by thought.

What was Nancy learning? She was discovering that there were different ways she could pay attention and know herself. If she thought about her body in her usual way, her mind would be filled with ideas and concepts and all their associations. Now she saw that she could focus on her body or any part of it, but as patterns of directly experienced sensations. Although she did not know it, she had shifted her mode of mind from doing to being as this experiment unfolded.

> **Direct sensing of the body turns up the volume on the body's messages and turns down the volume on mental chatter.**

This shift is particularly important to those of us who have struggled with chronic unhappiness because for us the thoughts that are so quick to jump in and take over are often negative and self-critical, and they pull us down into depression. The experience of inhabiting the body with full awareness without succumbing

THE NEW SCIENCE OF SENSATION

Even though the default mode network (DMN) wraps us up in habit (see page 44), we have other brain networks that are dedicated to exploring new perspectives. To do so, we need input from our senses. In fact, the distinction between sensing and responding is one of the most fundamental ways the brain is organized. Thousands of studies reveal that data from our senses land in the back half of the brain, leaving the front of the brain to figure out what to do with it. To recognize an object, for example, the visual cortex determines where edges start and end, how near or far the object is, and whether it is stationary or in motion. Once this input is decoded, the front of your brain can take over and label the object on the way to determining how relevant it is to you. Emotions follow the same pathway. They start out as sensory signals and are then quickly named and evaluated. It is easy to miss out on the early steps, when emotions show up as bodily sensations, because of strong tendencies to overthink. We wind up trying to figure out what to do about them, rather than just letting them be. *Direct sensing of the body turns down the volume on mental chatter and allows us to sense the body's messages more clearly.*

to the pull of our thoughts about the body can lead to a profoundly liberating change in our relationship to our bodies—and to life more generally.

In time and with practice, we can extend this little experiment with bringing mindfulness to our hands to the entire body. In the process, we may see a marked shift in our attention, away from living so much of our lives in our heads and toward letting our awareness take up residence in the whole of the body. In our mindfulness training programs, we begin to nurture such a shift through a meditation practice known as the "body scan."

The Body Scan

The body scan is a lying-down meditation practice we introduce in the very first session of our mindfulness programs and then ask people to practice daily for at least two weeks on their own at home. The body scan guides us in paying attention, directly and systematically, to each part of the body in turn. It encourages us to be in a more interested, intimate, and friendly relationship to the body in the present moment. It is sometimes challenging to bring attention to all the varied regions of the body in this way. For that reason, we use the breath to "carry" awareness into each part of the body, imagining, or sensing, that the breath can actually move throughout the body, bringing with it a direct, experiential sensing and knowing of the region of the body we are focusing on.

You might like to do this exercise yourself right now or later, using the instructions on Track 2 of the audio guidance available at *www.guilford.com/ williams3-materials*. Feel free to read the description on pages 103–105 first, but it's better to use the audio guidance when you come to practice the body scan.

A RELAXING MEDITATION?

As we see from the instructions for the body scan, the point of this practice is to be aware of your body as it is. It is not to achieve a state of relaxation. And yet deep states of relaxation often emerge, so much so that people sometimes find themselves falling asleep. Of course, if this happens, we often blame ourselves for not staying awake and compound our distress with a self-critical attitude. Alternatively we can see if it makes a difference to practice with eyes open or sitting up rather than lying down or to practice at a different time of day. We can also take a kindly attitude toward any feelings of sleepiness that do occur. And we can investigate what sleepiness feels like from the inside. In all these various ways, we gradually learn how to "fall awake" and stay awake while practicing meditation lying down, no matter how relaxed we do or don't get.

Jan found that she got so relaxed with the body scan that the sensations from the body gave her the impression of floating:

"At the end, I was so relaxed, it was as if my limbs and trunk weren't actually real. I know it might sound really strange, but it was wonderful, as if I was floating. It's very hard to describe. I think my breathing was a lot slower; I should think my heart was a lot slower. I just felt my whole body had sort of slowed down completely."

BODY SCAN MEDITATION

Track 2 of the audio files at *www.guilford.com/williams3-materials*

Preparation

1. Make yourself comfortable lying down on your back, in a place where you will feel warm and undisturbed. You can lie on a mat or rug on the floor or on your bed. Allow your eyes to close gently.

2. Take a few moments to get in touch with the movement of your breath and the sensations in your body. When you are ready, bring your awareness to the physical sensations in your body, especially to the sensations of touch or pressure where your body makes contact with the floor or bed. On each out-breath, allow yourself to sink a little deeper into the mat or bed.

3. To set the appropriate intention, remind yourself that this will be a time for "falling awake" rather than falling asleep. Remind yourself as well that the idea here is to be aware of your experience as it is unfolding, however it is. It is not to change the way you are feeling or to become more relaxed or calmer. The intention of this practice is to bring awareness to any and all sensations you are able to be aware of (or lack of sensation) as you focus your attention systematically on each part of the body in turn.

4. Now bring your awareness to the sensations in the belly, becoming aware of the changing patterns of sensations in the abdominal wall as the breath moves into the body and as it moves out of the body. Take a few minutes to feel the sensations as you breathe in and as you breathe out, as the belly rises on the in-breath and falls on the out-breath.

Moving Attention around the Body

5. Having connected with the sensations in the belly, now bring the focus or spotlight of your attention down the left leg, into the left foot, and all the way to the toes. Focus on each of the toes in turn, bringing a gentle, interested, affectionate attention to be with and investigate the quality of the sensations you find, perhaps noticing the sense of contact between the toes, a sense of tingling, warmth, perhaps numbness, whatever is here, perhaps even no sensations at all if that is the case. It is all okay. In fact, whatever you are experiencing is okay; it is what is here right now.

6. When you are ready, on an in-breath, feel or imagine the breath entering the lungs and then passing all the way down the body, through the left leg, to the toes of the left foot. On the out-breath, feel or imagine the breath coming all the way back up from the toes and the foot, right up through the leg and torso and out through the nose. As best you can, continue breathing in this way for a few breaths, breathing down into the toes on each in-breath and back out from the toes on each out-breath. It may be difficult to get the hang of this—just practice this "breathing into" as best you can, approaching it playfully.

7. Now, when you are ready, on an out-breath, let go of the toes and bring your awareness to the sensations in the bottom of your left foot—bringing a gentle, investigative awareness to the sole of the foot, the instep, the heel (noticing, for example, the sensations where the heel makes contact with the mat or bed). Experiment with "breathing with" any and all sensations—being aware of the breath in the background, as, in the foreground, you explore the sensations in the bottom of the foot.

8. Now allow the awareness to expand into the rest of the foot—to the ankle, the top of the foot, right into the bones and joints. Then take a deeper and more intentional breath in, directing it down into the whole of the left foot, and, as the breath lets go on the out-breath, let go of the left foot completely, allowing the focus of awareness to move into the lower left leg—the calf, shin, knee, and so forth, in turn.

9. Continue to scan the body, lingering for a time with each part of the body in turn: the left shin, the left knee, the left thigh; the right toes and then foot and ankle, the right lower leg, the right knee, the right thigh; the pelvic area—groin, genitals, buttocks, and hips; the lower back and the abdomen, the upper back and the chest and shoulders. Then we move to hands, usually doing both at the same time. We rest first with the sensations in the fingers and thumbs, the palms and the backs of both hands, the wrists, the lower arms and elbows, the upper arms; the shoulders again and the armpits; the neck; the face (jaw, mouth, lips, nose, cheeks, ears, eyes, forehead); and then the entirety of the head.

10. When you become aware of tension or of other intense sensations in a particular part of the body, you can "breathe in" to those sensations in the same way as for any others—using the in-breath to gently bring awareness right into the sensations, and, as best you can, have a sense of what happens in that region, if anything, as each breath lets go and releases on the out-breath.

When the Mind Wanders

11. The mind will inevitably wander away from the breath and the body from time to time. That is entirely normal. It is what minds do. When you notice it, gently acknowledge it, noticing where the mind has gone off to, and then gently return your attention to the part of the body you intended to focus on.

Ending

12. After you have scanned the whole body in this way, spend a few minutes being aware of a sense of the body as a whole and of the breath flowing freely in and out of the body.

13. It is also very important to remind yourself that if you, like many people, suffer from low-grade chronic sleep deprivation, since the body scan is done lying down, it is very easy to fall asleep. If you find yourself falling asleep, you might find it helpful to prop your head up with a pillow, open your eyes, or do the practice sitting up rather than lying down.

Jan also said it came as a great relief to enter a level of the mind that was not dominated by thinking. She said she was able to let go of all the mental clutter during the body scan and found it profoundly calming.

Why might we find it relaxing even though we are not purposely trying to relax? The body scan, like the breathing meditation described in Chapter 4, invites us to focus on relatively narrow aspects of our total experience in any given moment. Furthermore, it asks us to systematically shift from one locus of attention in the body to another over a fairly extended period of time. We might expect that the mind would become steadier through such a discipline over time and that we might feel more relaxed as a result. As long as Jan was "living in her head," and knowing her experience only indirectly, through thought, it was very difficult for her to focus her attention wholeheartedly. Thoughts themselves are ephemeral and fleeting, hardly present for an instant before they trigger associations and memories that carry us far from where we were only a moment ago. For this reason, thoughts do not provide the stability of focus the mind needs if it is to be steady and calm. By contrast, when we cultivate mindfulness, by paying attention to the detailed pattern of sensations in a particular part of the body in any and every moment, we have a vivid and accessible object to anchor our attention in each moment, even if its location is shifting over time as we move through the body. Just being able to focus on one thing at a time in this way allowed the rest of Jan's mind to settle, and she experienced a sense of calm, even though she was not looking for it.

Similarly, the nonstriving quality of mindfulness introduced in Chapter 4 fosters the development of peace and calm. There is no agenda other than to be awake, nowhere to get to, no special state to look out for or to try to attain. No matter what sensations we encounter when we practice the body scan—and that might include numbness or no sensation, or, for that matter, unpleasant or even painful sensations in certain regions—we allow them all to be just as they are, rather than trying to change them in any way. We are not trying to close the gap between the way things are and the way the driven-doing mind would like them to be. Instead, we are resting in our moment-by-moment experiencing of what is already here to be perceived, to be known directly, not through the intermediary of thought. You could say we are resting in the domain of being, in awareness itself. It's not hard to imagine that such an orientation toward our experience might be calming.

That said, it can be unhelpful for people to see the body scan as a form of relaxation training for the simple reason that it encourages old habits of mind to start up again. As with the breathing meditation in Chapter 4, we can inadvertently turn discovery into expectation and end up making relaxation the purpose and goal of the body scan: "This calm is what it's all about; this means I'm getting somewhere." This is precisely what Jan experienced. She had felt very relaxed, floating, wonderful. "But then, I think it was two days later, I could feel myself drifting off like that again. I remember thinking *Ah, here it is again. This is wonderful.* And as soon as I thought this, I could feel myself losing it, and I thought, *Oh, I want it to be like that again.* And then I was really disappointed. The last two or three times that I've listened to the audio, I found myself thinking beforehand, *Oh great, I hope I'm going to feel like that again.* And it hasn't happened."

Jan wanted to experience relaxation so badly that it escaped her, like a handful of dry sand grasped so tightly that it runs through the fingers. So what can we or Jan do at this point?

If we find the body scan peaceful and calming, we can simply be aware of these feelings experientially. To experience feelings is to know that they come and they go; they arise and they pass away. The point is to be here for them, to be directly aware of them as they are, whether pleasant, unpleasant, or neutral and barely noticeable.

Gradually, people discover for themselves the power of working in this way with whatever is arising in the body scan. It is the basis of a profound insight: when we stop trying to attain pleasant feelings, such feelings are more likely to emerge by themselves. With this insight may come another profound lesson: we *already* have the capacity to experience peace and happiness deep within ourselves. As we have said, we do not have to earn enough points to deserve it or hunt for it someplace else. We simply have to learn how to skillfully get out of our own way. Getting out of our own way allows the deep reservoirs of peace and happiness within us to reveal themselves so we may gain more ready access to them. For those of us who have been "fighting" unhappiness for much of our lives, this can be an enormously liberating change.

The invitation with the body scan and with all mindfulness practices is to let go of our expectations as far as it's possible for us at that moment. Expectations can become goals, which only get in the way of the experience we are having in this moment. But when we recognize that we are developing expectations, as Jan did, we can see how vulnerable we are to turning aspects of our experience into fixed goals—an important lesson in and of itself. It helps us learn to recognize when we are shifting into doing mode. By cultivating mindfulness in the body scan on a regular basis, Jan was beginning to recognize this pattern and found herself smiling at its antics.

When we stop trying to force pleasant feelings,
they are freer to emerge on their own.
When we stop trying to resist unpleasant feelings,
we may find that they can drift away by themselves.
When we stop trying to make *something* happen,
a whole world of fresh and unanticipated
experiences may become accessible to us.

MIND WANDERING: ANOTHER OPPORTUNITY TO RECOGNIZE DOING MODE

One of the most useful functions of the mind is to keep bringing up unfinished business so that goals that are important to us will not fall by the wayside. This little tickler system can keep us from missing a critical deadline or ensure that we patch up a damaged friendship that's important to us. But this function has a tendency to volunteer for duty when we don't need it, as Lauren found during her practice of the body scan.

Quite a lot had been happening in Lauren's family. Her partner's father, Phil, had recently fallen and broken his hip, and it had taken a lot of effort to figure out a way to get good care for him, given that all of his children and their partners worked full time. Lauren was focusing on sensations in her hip when she found her mind wandering.

"First I was sensing my hip," she said, "then I noticed myself thinking about its shape and remembering a picture of the hip in my biology textbook. Then I remembered Phil's broken hip—and I started to think about him in the hospital."

We can notice how the first step in the wanderings of Lauren's mind was relatively subtle; she made a shift from focusing on the *direct sensation* of the hip to *thinking about* the hip—from knowing through experience to knowing through ideas.

And once Pandora's box was opened, all the associations, memories, and other clutter of the doing mind rushed to the surface to take Lauren further and further from her intended focus: first to an association from her past, then to Phil, and from there to the image of him lying in his hospital bed. Her mind's meanderings did not end there:

"That made me think about Phil's sister. She said she'd take time off to look after him, but she hasn't. Then I was remembering a difficult phone call in which another member of the family said that she just couldn't cope with the parents anymore."

Once she had strayed from her intended focus on physical sensations in the body, Lauren's attention shifted to the unfinished business of caregiving and families. At some stage (she wasn't sure when) she nodded off to sleep for a few minutes.

At first Lauren was angry when her mind continued to wander. But, after practicing the body scan for about two weeks, she noticed that something was changing in her. "Before," she said, "I would get into a tizzy and start throwing mental pots and pans about the place—just in my mind, you understand. I'd think and think: *Well, no one cares; I'm the only one that knows what to do about Phil and how to look after him, and if they can't do it, then they can stay away for all I care.* Well, the pots and pans I was throwing in my mind only hurt *me*, because no one else saw them being thrown. Now I can feel the stress in my body, but I'm neither running away from it nor getting upset about being upset."

Lauren found that, when her mind wandered off, it was more effective and appropriate to simply smile to herself in recognition of it and just gently bring it back to where she had intended it to be rather than to berate herself. Furthermore, she said that coming back to the level of sensations allowed her to be in touch with, and even "feel" the stress of her life, but without overreacting.

NO SUCH THING AS A BAD MEDITATION

Whether we've come to expect the relaxation or calm that may accompany the body scan or we tend to scold ourselves for letting our minds wander, it's easy to attach goals to meditation and start to think of a particular session as "good" or "bad" or as "working" or "not working." Because of the aversion we feel for unpleasant emotion, we may also be tempted, if we felt impatient throughout, restless, uncomfortable, itchy or irritable, cold or hot, or in pain, to say we had a "bad" meditation. We may never want to do the body scan again, because, obviously, the meditation didn't "work." Something was wrong: maybe we blame the audio guidance or the teacher or the method, or we think of ourselves as failures. And if we also imagine that meanwhile other people are having wonderful experiences with the body scan, we will just have one more reason to think we're failing.

There is no such thing as failing at meditation, as long as we are mindful of our experience, whatever it is. In fact, this is precisely why the body scan is so powerful. It gives us opportunity after opportunity to rest in or return to the being mode, with its direct experiential knowing, even in the presence of strong emotion, thoughts, or sensations. Like all the other meditation practices, the body scan becomes a laboratory for our own learning and growing—*learning* not to get stuck in self-perpetuating cycles of preoccupation and unhappiness, *growing* into a greater intimacy and comfort with ourselves. The things that come up from moment to moment in the body scan all become our teachers to further this learning and this growing, whether they appear as pleasant, unpleasant, or neutral.

> There is no such thing as a "good" meditation or a "bad" meditation as long as we are mindfully aware and see clearly what is unfolding in the present moment.

The body scan is aimed at freeing us from the suffering and mental anguish that arises through wanting things to be different from the way they are in this moment. In the body scan, as in life itself, we are in a much stronger, freer position if we can let go of the desire to feel calm—or enlightened or at peace or filled with joy—and instead can learn to be present with whatever we are feeling right now.

This might mean recognizing tension or restlessness in certain regions of the body and letting them be as they are, instead of starting a mental harangue about why we're feeling such stress.

It might mean noticing an overall sense of tiredness but not wearing ourselves out with exhortations to perk up and get going.

It might mean feeling a glimmering of peace or joy under layers of moodiness, tension, or irritation and just knowing it's there, rather than digging frantically to drag it to the surface and demand that it makes us feel better right this minute.

Mindful Awakening in the Morning

Let's return to where we began: feeling an unpleasant heaviness and fatigue on waking in the morning. For many of us, dealing with this feeling can be quite difficult. Of course we would rather not experience such feelings. But here is where the practice of the body scan may be of real use. If we have practiced the body scan for even a few days, we will have begun relating to the body as it is and not as we may wish it were. In the body scan, we discover the possibility of approaching things from a fresh perspective, and this becomes applicable at all times, even when we don't have time to do an extended body scan.

So, on waking, how might we approach the situation differently? We will be able to recognize the early warning signs of what might become a vicious cycle and begin to practice inhabiting the being mode of mind. We

WHY STICK WITH THE BODY SCAN?

A lot of importance is attached to the body scan in our mindfulness training programs; from the very beginning the people participating in these programs spend forty-five minutes a day on this practice, six days a week, for at least the first two weeks, even when, as often happens, they may not feel much immediate benefit. If you find yourself struggling with keeping up the practice, you might like to follow the advice we give to those attending our training programs: just do it as best you can and stay in the process whether you think it is "working" or not. The practice itself winds up revealing new possibilities if you just stay with it. *Why?*

- Because the body scan provides a wonderful arena to cultivate a new, experiential way of knowing.

- Because the body scan offers us the opportunity to reconnect with our bodies, which play a key role in the experience and expression of emotion.

- Because mindful awareness of sensations in our bodies can uncouple the links between body sensations and thinking that keep the cycle of rumination and unhappiness going.

- Because the body scan teaches us to bring wise and openhearted attention to parts of the body even when they are the site of intensely unpleasant sensations—a skill that can then be generalized to other aspects of our lives.

On the horizon, then, is the possibility of freeing ourselves from some of our most limiting self-imposed constraints on happiness and well-being.

will focus our attention directly on our body sensations and rest in the aware-ness of them as they are. This allows us to be with the uncomfortable sensa-tions without trying to avoid them or making them worse through thinking about them. Even in the very earliest stages of the body scan practice, this alternative to doing mind can have an impact on something as common and mundane as early morning weariness. That sense of heaviness is greatly increased by negative thoughts. But mindfulness in the same situation—bringing a gentle and compassionate awareness to the bodily sensations themselves, without trying to change them, and letting go of thoughts about them or about ourselves, or *about* anything—can be immensely energizing.

Once we have some experience with the body scan, we can bring this kind of awareness to bear in a matter of moments. We can even scan the body for one in-breath and one out-breath or just breathe with the body as a whole for five minutes or so, or even a minute or two, before getting out of bed.

It might just change our whole day.

Part III

Transforming Unhappiness

Six

Reconnecting with Our Feelings—Those We Like, Those We Don't Like, and Those We Don't Know We Have

John was driving home from work, held up in a line of cars at a stop light, when a truck in front of him backed up, hitting the front of his car. It didn't do much damage, but enough for John to know that he'd have to call the insurance company. Even worse, the truck driver had denied he was backing up. He said that John had just driven into him from behind. John drove home in a quiet fury. He was tense, his face was red, his blood pressure was up, he was frowning. When he arrived home, he slumped into a chair and decided not to worry about the car until tomorrow. That made him feel better. He picked up the mail. The first letter was from his bank, asking if he would call to discuss something concerning his pension payments. John rose from the chair, thumped on the table, and stormed out of the house.

Only later, once he and his partner had talked about it, was it clear to John that his tension over the car had spilled into his reaction to the (otherwise innocuous) letter. John's partner said they had been able to tell he was tense just by looking at him. His whole body had seemed tight, and his posture was that of someone who was fed up. John himself had no idea that he was still feeling so bad. He looked surprised when his partner asked him if he was feeling better and denied having any lingering feelings about the accident or the letter. He simply brushed off both as passing annoyances, saying he was fine, with a tight smile that looked more like a grimace.

John was completely out of touch with the signals his body was sending him—not just on this one occasion but as a rule. As a result, he didn't really notice all of his emotional reactions—at least not before they had pulled his mood downward. By then it was too late to take timely action to deal with them. Not only that, but John's overreaction to the bank's letter was a direct result of the tension that was lingering following his encounter with the truck driver. His lack of awareness meant that the state of his mind was controlled by his body and emotions to an extent that would have alarmed him. As we saw in Chapters 2 and 5, the state of our bodies supplies important information to the mind, and, if we are unaware of it, this can powerfully affect our judgments, thoughts, and feelings. Frowning, for instance, makes us judge our experiences more negatively. By the same token, John's tight body and grimacing expression kindled a frustration that fed into his reaction to the bank's letter.

His unawareness of the full range of his emotional and physical responses was a direct result of his efforts to avoid feelings he didn't want.

Why We Tune Out

As we discussed in Chapter 2, it is understandable that we make an enemy of our emotions if we've experienced painful moods and feelings in the past. We react to our own unhappiness as if it were a threat, and when we do so, the brain's avoidance system is triggered. Not only do we damp down approach-related behaviors, such as curiosity, engagement, and goodwill, but the mind is also driven to avoid even its own productions by walling them off, suppressing them, numbing out, or, in one way or another, pretending that they are not around even when they are. The effect is not only to disconnect us from negative or uncomfortable feelings and body sensations, but possibly to mute our ability to feel anything, positive or negative. We handicap ourselves in dealing effectively with unhappiness and reinforce the sense that, somehow, we are out of touch with the full experience of being alive but don't know exactly why.

This attempt to avoid our own emotions, our thoughts, our feelings, and our body sensations is called *experiential avoidance*. Not surprisingly, it can become a habit. Who wouldn't tune out feelings and body sensations if the news on this frequency had been too unpleasant too often? But pretending some feeling isn't actually here is like hearing a strange noise from your car engine while driving along the freeway and dealing with it by turning up the volume on the car radio. It works pretty well to blank out the noise, but is not too effective in preventing the engine from seizing up ten miles down the road. Psychologist Steve Hayes and his colleagues concluded from a review of more than one hundred research studies that many forms of emotional disturbance are the result of unhealthy efforts to escape and avoid emotions—that is, the result of experiential avoidance. If we try to wall off bodily sensations, thoughts, and feelings that are part and parcel of our emotional experience, then psychologically our mental "engines" are highly likely to seize up as well!

In the long run, experiential avoidance simply does not work as a way to deal with unwanted and unpleasant feelings. Although we might not be aware of them, the unpleasant feelings are still with us, and they still trigger habitual reactions that can turn passing feelings of unpleasantness into persistent suffering. Unless we are aware of them, unpleasant feelings will directly and indirectly influence our attitudes and judgments in ways that only perpetuate our unhappiness. *Unless we are aware.* There's the issue. When "tuning out" has become a habit, how can we learn to "tune back in" without becoming overwhelmed? It is helpful to know that an aspect of our inner experience can help. We call it the "internal barometer."

THE INTERNAL BAROMETER

When looking for a new place to live, we often spend many hours visiting potential homes. Have you ever come upon a house or an apartment that looked perfect online—it had the number of rooms you need, more than adequate square footage, excellent amenities, and a great neighborhood—until you visited it? As soon as you walked through the door, you knew it was not the place for you. You may not have been able to say why. It was just an intuition. It was conscious—you were very aware of it—yet not expressible in words. It was just, somehow, a readout of your directly sensed gut-level evaluation of the situation. It may even have been so strong that you just wanted to get out as quickly as possible.

Our feelings may have many dimensions, but underneath and underpinning them all is a single scale in the mind that simply registers experience as "positive," "neutral," or "negative." It is as if this capacity functions as an internal barometer. Just as a real barometer provides a continuous readout of atmospheric pressure, this internal barometer provides a readout of the "internal atmosphere" of our experience in each moment. But just as we need to *read* the barometer to gain information about the weather, we will need to read (and, if necessary, learn how to read) this internal barometer by becoming more aware of what we are really feeling from moment to moment. In this way we have the possibility to act more appropriately and with greater balance of mind, particularly in very trying situations.

We do this by learning to attend more closely to the chain of our reactions to any object, person, place, or event we encounter. If we do so, we'll discover that there is an instinctive sense of the experience as pleasant, unpleasant, or neutral. If an experience registers as pleasant, the chain of reactions will tend to go in one direction, at the end of which we may become aware of wanting to prolong the experience. If an experience registers as unpleasant, the chain of reactions will cascade in another direction, at the end of which we may become aware of wanting it to go away or to escape from it. Often most of this is completely automatic and goes on beneath the surface of awareness.

> Each of us has an internal monitor of experience that registers whether something is pleasant, unpleasant, or neutral. It can act as an early warning system. When we learn to read it, we can free ourselves from knee-jerk aversion and, in turn, rumination.

If we actually *practice* bringing awareness to the chain of reactions to particular moments and circumstances, we have an excellent opportunity, each time we do so, to break the strong link between these basic "gut feelings" and the totally automatic and also largely unconscious reactions that follow so rapidly on their heels, and in particular the reaction we have described as aversion. Since "unpleasantness" is common to and underneath all negative emotions—sadness, anger, disgust, and anxiety—we have the chance to develop a generic "early warning system" for all uncomfortable emotions, whatever form they take as they emerge into consciousness. By tuning in with great sensitivity to the messages of the internal barometer, we may recognize any unpleasant feelings that we have previously screened out, *as they are actually arising*. Bringing them into awareness weakens their influence over our mind and enables us to respond to them in ways that do not evoke or perpetuate aversion and make spiraling into depression more likely.

What is the most reliable way to tune in to this early warning system? We hinted at it in Chapter 5. By bringing awareness to the body in a certain way, we can discover and make wise use of our own internal barometer.

Opening Up New Possibilities

To accomplish this, we need an effective way to tune in to body sensations and feelings so we know, directly and immediately, our intuitive evaluation of any moment. That will give us a chance to respond to a particular situation in ways that are more effective than our habitual, automatic emotional reactions.

For example, if a fleeting memory makes us feel suddenly sad or unhappy, we may not need to know what aspect of the memory triggered the emotion. The memory itself, or the emotion it evokes, will be registered as "unpleasant," and it is this gut sense of unpleasantness that fuels the chain reaction that ensues. This might once have been the start of a downward spiral, but it doesn't have to be. For *we can transform a cascade of reactions into a series of choice points*.

The moment in which we notice aversion emerging in response to our identifying some event (such as a sad feeling) as unpleasant becomes a defining moment, a critical point at which mindfulness can open up new possibilities. For one thing, by bringing a friendly nonjudgmental awareness right in close to the body sensations that accompany the unhappiness, we can immediately make wiser use of the information implicit in the sensations and feelings themselves. Eventually we will discover ways of responding mindfully to the unhappiness itself, as it is felt in the body. This enormously increases the likelihood that it will either dissolve on the spot or dissipate more gradually in its own good time.

SAD MOOD INHIBITS SENSATIONS

Why open awareness to directly sensed experience of the body? Because all our efforts when we are depressed tend to be devoted to ruminative brooding as the daydreaming of the default mode network (DMN) turns negative.

We can see this by using a brain scanner to explore what happens when participants watch sad films. The sadness activates the DMN at the expense of sensory processing. That is, in some people, the DMN actively shuts down the processing of sensation.

What happens when people watch sad films in an fMRI scanner and are then followed for two years to see who gets depressed and who stays well? Farb et al. asked this exact question. What they weren't sure about was whether the DMN's dominance over sensation would leave people more vulnerable to depression. They found that sadness did indeed shut down sensory processing and that a higher-than-average intensity of sensory shutdown made a person twenty-five times more likely to become depressed than someone who experienced less intense levels of shutdown.

A hopeful aspect of this work is that the DMN activity tended to quiet down following eight weeks of mindfulness-based cognitive therapy. Relying on this region to respond to sadness with fixing, thinking, and planning made relapse more likely, whereas learning to reduce its influence through mindfulness or curiosity was associated with resilience.

We may now begin to see how opening our awareness to our directly sensed experience of the body can reconnect us with emotions that we may have been avoiding. For many of us, it may be difficult at first to differentiate between that first perception of an "unpleasant" quality within the experience and the downstream reaction of aversion, because they are likely to be experienced as a fused whole. That is not necessarily a problem because we can always just take it one step at a time. First, we may be able to be aware of the whole "fused" ensemble as a feeling of overall contraction somewhere in the body that itself feels somewhat unpleasant. Second, having recognized the contraction at the level of sensation and become a little more familiar with it, we can begin to recognize the unpleasant feeling/aversion ensemble more and more clearly. This is a great step forward. Then, by practicing meditations that are specifically focused on refining our awareness of the body (such as the body scan and the practices described in this chapter), it can become easier to detect the unpleasant quality in the feeling *before* it triggers aversion. Finally, and little by little, we may begin to notice that they are distinct—the unpleasantness registered first, followed by the "get me out of here" reaction of aversion, which is also then registered as unpleasant, and so the cycle continues.

It is helpful to know that the most easily recognized expressions of aversion in the body are feelings of contraction in the shoulders or lower back, a tightening of the forehead, a clenching of the jaw, and a tightening of the belly. We have these fight-or-flight reactions whether we're trying to escape from a tiger or from our own feelings. Like John, however, we often stop noticing these aversive physiological reactions when the tiger is inside us and has been with us for quite some time with no evident plans to vacate the premises.

So, taking it one step at a time, how can we become more aware of the "ensemble" we have described, the body sensations that will reveal the fusion of the initial barometer reading "unpleasant" and the cascade of habitual reactions that follow it? We have already started, for there is an infinite number of opportunities each time we practice the body scan (Chapter 5). Can we be aware of feelings of unpleasantness or pleasantness and their immediate manifestation as sensations in the body moment by moment? As we continue in that practice, we naturally become more familiar with the feelings expressed not only in particular regions of the body, but also in a sense of the body as a whole, held in awareness, as we do at the end of each body scan.

The exercises in this chapter will help us expand and deepen our capacity to discern the whole domain of our intuitive evaluations of experience as pleasant, unpleasant, or neutral, and how these express themselves in the body. This will involve, among other things, deepening our familiarity and comfort level with our awareness of the body as a unified whole and how it can help us read that vital internal barometer so we know which way the interior winds are blowing. But first we must explore some questions concerning the *quality* of our awareness and our underlying motivations and how significant these might be in the practices described in this chapter and, for that matter, in all of the mindfulness practices we are developing.

The Mouse in the Maze

Do you remember the puzzle books that we got when we were children? There might be connect-the-dots puzzles and find-the-differences puzzles. No doubt whoever was looking after us at the time hoped it would take many quiet hours for us to join the dots or find the differences between two almost identical pictures. Sometimes there'd be a maze—a labyrinth—and our task would be to draw a way out without taking the pencil off the page.

Some years ago psychologists used a similar maze puzzle in an intriguing experiment with college students. A cartoon mouse was shown trapped inside a picture of a maze, and the task was to help the mouse find the way out. There were two different versions of the task. One was positive, approach-oriented; the other was negative or avoidance-oriented. In the positive condition, there was a piece of Swiss cheese lying outside the maze, in front of a mouse hole. In the negative condition, the maze was exactly the same, but instead of the Swiss cheese feast at the finish, an owl hovered above the maze, ready to swoop down and capture the mouse in its talons at any moment.

The maze takes less than two minutes to complete, and all the students who took part in the experiment solved their maze. But the contrast in the *aftereffects* of working on different versions of the maze was striking. When the participants later took a test of creativity, those who had helped their mouse avoid the owl turned in scores that were 50 percent lower than the scores of students who had helped their mouse find the cheese. The state of mind elicited by attending to the owl had resulted in a lingering sense of caution, avoidance, and vigilance for things going wrong. This mind-state in turn weakened creativity, closed down options, and reduced the students' flexibility in responding to the next task.

> **Goodwill and warm curiosity toward our feelings will put us in greater touch with the full experience of each moment of our lives.**

This experiment tells us something very important: the same action (even something as slight as solving a simple maze puzzle) has different consequences depending on whether it is done to move toward something we welcome (activating the brain's approach system) or to avoid something negative (activating the brain's avoidance system). In the maze experiment, aversion was triggered by something as minor as the sight of a cartoon owl. It led to reductions in exploratory, creative behaviors. This is dramatic evidence that the avoidance system can narrow the focus of our lives, even when triggered by a purely symbolic threat. Moreover, this experiment points to the critical importance of the kind of motivation that we bring to the cultivation of mindfulness in our practice. If we can infuse our attention to our bodily experience with the approach qualities of interest, curiosity, warmth, and goodwill, then not only will we be in greater touch with sensations and feelings in each moment, we also will be directly countering any effects of aversion and avoidance that may be present. As with so much of what we are learning to do, cultivating wholesome and kind intention and motivation is just as much a part of meditation practice as learning how to focus our attention in particular ways.

Mindful Yoga

In the practice that follows, which builds on the work of refining bodily awareness that we started in the body scan, we bring our attention to the range of sensations and feelings that arise in our bodies as we go through a ten-minute sequence of gentle standing yoga stretches. In the practice of mindful movement, be sure to take special care if you have any physical problems that limit your movement. Consult your physician or physical therapist if you are unsure (see also page 234). You might like to do this practice now, or as soon as you can, following the guidance on audio Track 3 (*www.guilford.com/williams3-materials*). You can also read the instructions in the box on pages 124–125, but it's better to use the audio guidance when you come to practice mindful standing yoga.

In the full mindfulness-based cognitive therapy (MBCT) program, this introductory exposure is followed by a sitting meditation and alternated day by day with a more extended sequence of mindful movements, stretches, and

MINDFUL STANDING YOGA

Track 3 of the audio files at *www.guilford.com/williams3-materials*

Preparation

1. First, we stand in bare feet or socks with our feet about hips-width apart, with the knees unlocked so that the legs can bend slightly and with the feet parallel (it's actually unusual to stand with the feet like this, and this, itself, can generate some novel bodily sensations).

2. Next we remind ourselves of the intention of this practice: to become aware, as best we can, of physical sensations and feelings throughout the body as we engage in a series of gentle stretches, honoring and investigating the limitations of our body in every moment, as best we can letting go of any tendency to push beyond our limits or to compete with either ourselves or others.

Moving

3. Then, on an in-breath, we slowly and mindfully raise our arms out to the sides, parallel to the floor, and then, after breathing out, we continue on the next in-breath raising them, slowly and mindfully, until our hands meet above our heads, all the while perhaps feeling the tension in the muscles as they work to lift the arms and then maintain them in the stretch.

4. Then, letting the breath move in and out freely at its own pace, we continue to stretch upward, the fingertips gently pushing toward the sky, the feet firmly grounded on the floor, as we feel the stretch in the muscles and joints of the body all the way from the feet and legs up through the back, shoulders, into the arms, hands, and fingers.

5. We maintain that stretch for a time, breathing freely in and out, noticing any changes in the sensations and feelings in the body with the breath as we continue to hold the stretch. Of course, this might include a sense of increasing tension or discomfort, and if so, opening to that as well.

6. At a certain point, when we are ready, we slowly, very slowly, on an out-breath, allow the arms to come back down. We lower them slowly, with the wrists bent so that the fingers point upward and the palms are pushing outward (again, an unusual position) until the arms come back to rest alongside the body, hanging from the shoulders.

7. We then allow the eyes to close gently and focus attention on the movements of the breath and the sensations and feelings throughout the body as we stand here, perhaps noticing the contrast in the physical sense of release (and often relief) associated with returning to a neutral stance.

8. We continue now by mindfully stretching each arm and hand up in turn, as if we were picking fruit from a tree when it was just out of reach, with full awareness of the sensations throughout the body, and of the breath; see what happens to the extension of the hand and to the breath if you lift the opposite heel off the floor while stretching up.

9. After this sequence, now slowly and mindfully raise both arms up high, keeping them parallel to each other, and then allow the body to bend to the left, with the hips going over to the right, forming a big crescent that extends in a sideways curve from the feet right through the torso, the arms, the hands, and the fingers. Then come back to standing on an in-breath, and then on an out-breath, slowing bending over, forming a curve in the opposite direction.

10. Once you have returned to standing in a neutral position with the arms alongside the body, you can play with rolling the shoulders while letting the arms dangle passively, first raising the shoulders upward toward the ears as far as they will go, then backward as if you were attempting to draw the shoulder blades together, then letting them drop down completely, then squeezing the shoulders together in front of the body as far as they will go, as if you were trying to touch them together with the arms passive and dangling. Continue "rolling" through these various positions as smoothly and mindfully as you can, with the arms dangling all the while, first in one direction, and then in the opposite direction, in a forward and backward "rowing" motion.

11. Then, once you have rested in a neutral standing posture again, play with slowly and mindfully rolling the head around to whatever degree you feel comfortable with it, and very gently, as if drawing a circle with the nose in midair, allowing the circling to move gently in one direction and then the other.

Ending

12. And finally, at the end of this sequence of movements, we remain still for a while, in a standing or sitting posture, and tune in to the sensations from the body.

postures based on hatha yoga practiced as a form of meditation in its own right. Because, to begin with, it is not easy to remember this sequence, we guide ourselves through one position after another, using detailed instructions from an audio track. If you wish to follow this longer sequence, there is audio guidance at Track 9, narrated by Zindel Segal (*www.guilford.com/ williams3-materials*).

The mouse-in-the-maze experiment reminds us of the crucial importance of the spirit in which we approach this practice. We invite ourselves to explore what is going on in our bodies in the same way that we investigated eating the raisin, bringing an openhearted awareness to whatever is available to be experienced from moment to moment. For this to happen, we will need to be aware of the habits we might harbor of avoiding certain kinds of experiences altogether, especially if they have an unpleasant quality to them. Unpleasant sensations will certainly arise at times and in various places in the body, especially while doing mindful yoga. These now become perfect opportunities for exploring how unpleasantness is related to aversion. So the challenge of each moment in the standing yoga is to purposefully experience the body just as it is moment by moment, with openness and interest, as if for the first time, and that includes sensing and gently exploring its limits in any given stretch or posture.

For instance, we can begin by recognizing the various sensations in the body for what they are, *as* sensations that arise and pass away. To do this, we will need to break through the screen of any fear-laden thoughts or expectations that might be present. Let's say we deliberately hold a stretch or a posture a little longer than feels comfortable and begin to experience some discomfort in the shoulders or back. The challenge is to put out the welcome mat for these sensations as we hold them in awareness and recognize their unpleasant quality. Can we notice the impulse to instantly label the sensations as "pain" or the whole experience as pure "torture"?

By turning *toward* discomfort and unpleasantness and by intentionally embracing them in awareness when they do arise, we are expanding the heart qualities of openness and goodwill in ourselves. By cultivating awareness in this way, we are weakening our tendency to avoid internal experiences we don't like. At the same time, we are also weakening our unconscious reliance on the doing mode, which, when fear-based, only entangles us in persistent unhappiness. Some people find it helpful to hone and deepen their awareness by silently inquiring "What is this?" as they attend to their experience.

Physical movements and stretching offer many opportunities to bring a spirit of gentleness, kindness, and compassion to ourselves, rather than pushing beyond our limits or being critical and judgmental of our "performance."

> **Gently asking "What is this?" when we encounter an unpleasant experience keeps the mind from leaping in with "I hate this—get me out of here!"**

RESPONDING TO THE YOGA

People respond differently to the practices we are describing, but many find these yoga stretches enormously helpful. For anyone who has a hard time with maintaining physical stillness over extended time periods, such as in the body scan, the mindful yoga can often be especially effective. These postures, movements, and stretches readily ground us in the here and now, allowing us to feel fully present with our bodies and more awake to our wider experience of the moment.

Moving and stretching, like walking, often provide "louder" body sensations than either the meditation on the breath or the body scan meditation. As such, they can sometimes provide an easier focus on which to gather our attention and open to our experience. Furthermore, the stretching of muscles that may be habitually tensed in a chronic state of aversion can free us from emotions we may not know we are even harboring and in which we have nevertheless gotten stuck.

As with all the other practices, the awareness we cultivate in the mindful yoga is available to us in all our moments. Using the body to ground us in awareness during the course of the day can be as simple as becoming mindful of our posture or of any movement, large or small. This doesn't actually take any more time than being out of touch with our body and moving automatically and without awareness. Say we are reaching for something. We are doing it anyway. There's nothing extra we have to do. We simply bring attention to the body sensations in the region that is moving and the regions that are not moving. We can train ourselves to be here, right now, inhabiting the body with full awareness. Whatever is going on in our mind or body, our internal barometer is always here for us if we choose to read it.

Doing so gives us far greater choice in terms of what happens in the very next moment. This in itself adds a new degree of freedom to our relationship to our interior experience.

Widening Attention around the Breath

In addition to using the practice of mindful yoga to ground us in the body, we can deepen our awareness in ways that can help us tune in to the signals of our internal barometer. One very powerful one is to extend the practice of mindfulness of the breath that we explored in Chapter 4 to include a sense of the body as a whole. You might like to experiment with this practice before reading further, following the audio guidance on Track 5 of the recording available at *www.guilford.com/williams3-materials*. As with all the practices we are exploring, remember to bring the same quality of openheartedness to each moment as best you can, directly sensing body sensations and feelings *as* sensations and feelings.

New dimensions of the experiences of both pain (physical and emotional) and suffering and the potential for embracing them and understanding them differently become available to us when we give ourselves over to the present moment and let go of all thoughts of the future and the past at just those moments of highest intensity. You might experiment with this shift in motivation and awareness even for brief moments whenever physical or emotional intensity arises in the meditation practice. Just getting one toe in the water for even the briefest of moments, if that is all you can manage at a certain moment, rather than jumping into the pool, can be profoundly revealing and potentially healing.

MARIA'S STORY

Maria was cleaning up after a visit from her two children. They were in their mid-twenties and had left home for work and college some years before. Many of their possessions were still around the house as reminders that they would always be welcomed here. They had left that morning to get their train after a weekend celebrating their mother's fiftieth birthday; their noise and laughter faded as they disappeared around the corner of the road. Maria

SITTING MEDITATION:
MINDFULNESS OF THE BREATH AND BODY

Track 5 of the audio files at *www.guilford.com/williams3-materials*

1. Practice mindfulness of the breath, as described earlier (pages 77–78), for ten minutes in an erect and dignified sitting posture, whether in a chair or on the floor.

2. When you feel you have settled to some degree into feeling the breath moving in and out of your body at the belly or at the nostrils, intentionally allow the field of awareness to expand around the breath to include as well a sense of the various sensations throughout the body, whatever they are, and a sense of the body as a whole sitting and breathing. You may even find you get a sense of the breath moving throughout the body.

3. If you choose, include together with this wider sense of the body as a whole, and of the breath moving in and out of the body, awareness of the more local, particular patterns of physical sensations that arise where the body makes contact with the floor, chair, cushion, or stool—the sensations of touch, pressure, or contact of the feet or knees with the floor, the buttocks with whatever is supporting them, the hands where they rest on the thighs or together in the lap. As best you can, hold all these sensations, together with the sense of the breath and of the body as a whole, in a wide and spacious awareness.

4. Of course, in all likelihood, you will find the mind wandering repeatedly away from the breath and body sensations. Keep in mind that this is a natural tendency of the mind and is in no way a mistake or a sign of failure or "not doing it right." As we have noted before, whenever you notice that your attention has drifted away from sensations in the body, you might want to let it register that to be aware of that fact means that you are already back and awake to what is going on in the mind. In that very moment, it can be useful to gently note what was on your mind ("thinking," "planning," "remembering") and then to reestablish your attention on the breath sensations and a sense of the body as a whole.

5. As best you can, resting in a gentle attending to the actuality of the field of sensations throughout the body from moment to moment, and being aware of any feelings of pleasantness, unpleasantness, or neutrality as they arise.

6. The longer the session continues, the more you may experience sensations arising that are particularly intense in one region of your body or another, perhaps in the back or in the knees or in the shoulders. With greater intensity of sensations, especially if they feel unpleasant and uncomfortable, you may find that your attention is repeatedly drawn to them and away from your intended focus on the breath or the body as a whole. In such moments, rather than shifting your posture (although you are always free to do that, of course), you might experiment even briefly with intentionally bringing the focus of attention right into the region of greatest intensity and, as best you can, exploring with gentle and wise attention the detailed pattern of sensations there—what, precisely, are the qualities of the sensations; where, exactly, are they located; do they vary over time or shift around in the body from one place to another? This exploration is undertaken in the realm of sensing and feeling, rather than through thinking. Again, as best you can, opening to feeling whatever is already here to be felt, allowing yourself to know what you are feeling via directly experiencing it. As in the body scan, you may play with using the breath as a vehicle to carry awareness into such regions of intensity, "breathing in" to them, and out from them.

7. Notice how much "pain" can be created out of discomfort through the thoughts about such discomfort—especially thoughts about how long it is going to last. So, whenever you find yourself "carried away" by the intensity of physical sensations, or in any other way, as best you can, reconnect with the here and now by refocusing attention on the movements of the breath or on a sense of the body as a whole sitting in a balanced and dignified posture. In this way, you may find you are able, even in the midst of the intensity of sensation, to be grounded in the present moment.

would have to set off for work soon, but she thought she'd start a bit of laundry and clean one of the bedrooms. As she went into her son's room, she felt a sense of sadness and loneliness. "No," she said, "I cannot be sentimental; I've got to be strong. It's silly to feel sad." The moment passed; she took the sheets off the bed, picked up the wastepaper basket, and went downstairs.

Maria had gotten into the habit of dealing with any difficult emotion in this way; it is the way she had coped with a great deal of stress in her life. This strategy had seemed to work well, but it now meant that she was cut off from her feelings. She was afraid of experiencing any emotion lest it overwhelm her. She had begun to feel that she lived "in parallel" to herself and to those she loved. She always felt a little cut off, never really engaging with others without being self-conscious and feeling that she was acting out a part. What she noticed most was that she was constantly tired, exhausted for no good reason.

At some level she felt that, if she ever started crying, she wouldn't be able to stop—that she would cry for the whole world, for things and for people she had lost in her life, for her wrong decisions, for her lost children, for her unfulfilled ambitions. She would embarrass herself and let herself down; it would be shameful, uncontrollable. To enter the dangerous, uncharted territory of emotion was something she had learned to avoid a long time ago.

Some weeks earlier, Maria had enrolled in our mindfulness program. She had enjoyed the body scan and the yoga, though she found the

---

BREATHING *INTO*

The practice of expanding our attention around the breath to include a wider awareness of the body as a whole in the sitting meditation will provide many opportunities to refine the skills of "breathing into" that we described when we discussed the body scan in the last chapter (pages 103–105). When we shift from focusing primarily on the body as a whole, with the breath in the background, to focusing our attention *right into* the area of most intense physical sensations, there is much to discover. Although our attention may be drawn to the general area of intensity (as if the mind were shouting "Hey, look at this!"), our habit of trying to avoid any negative experience may offer some resistance to actually bringing awareness *right into* the most intense physical sensations and feelings, the epicenter, as it were, of our discomfort. "Breathing into" can offer a powerful antidote to experiential avoidance. The breath can be a vehicle carrying a gentle yet penetrating awareness into the region of intensity. We sense or imagine the breath, as it moves into the body, continuing its movement until it enters the very core of the region of intensity, carrying awareness with it.

If the intensity of the sensations becomes overwhelming, we can stabilize our attention through a complementary practice, *breathing with,* in which we hold awareness of the intensity together with awareness of the whole of the breath moving into and out of the body somewhat in the background.

BREATHING *WITH*

Widening the field of awareness, whether to our bodies or to other aspects of our experience, is sometimes difficult because there is so much going on: in our lives, our minds, and our bodies. We are virtually bombarded with stimuli inwardly and outwardly at all times except for, perhaps, deep sleep. How, in this situation, do we combine stability of mind with a wider awareness? One way is to take advantage of the obvious but remarkable fact that whatever we experience in our lives is always (and always has been) experienced with the activity of the breath in the background. This means that, if we choose, we can seamlessly weave awareness of the breath in with awareness of any other aspect of our experience. And by doing so, we reconnect in that moment with our capacity to steady the mind, that capacity we were developing earlier as we laid the foundations for mindfulness practice by focusing on the movements of the breath alone. We call this practice "breathing with." By including an awareness of the breath "in the background" as we focus on any experience, we can steady the mind, and so attend more easily to our actual experience in any moment.

For example, if you were to put on a piece of music right now, you would probably find that after focusing your attention on the music for a while, your mind would begin to wander. As an experiment now or some other time, you might like to see if you can pay attention to the music and also focus, in the background, on the breath as it moves in and out of your body. Try this for a few minutes, perhaps alternating the focus, first listening to the music alone and then also including attention to the breath in the background. It may take some trial and error to find the most comfortable way to do this. In particular, it may take a while to strike the right balance between the primary focus, the music, in the foreground and the steadying influence of the breath in the background. But many find the effort worthwhile because it offers us a very versatile way to steady the mind in complex and difficult situations. In particular, it can be an invaluable ally and support in our intention to expand the focus of awareness to the whole domain of felt bodily experience, when, as may often happen, this requires us to turn toward and face intense physical sensations and unpleasant feelings.

meditation on the breath very difficult. Her mind kept wandering, so she did not feel settled in the practice and didn't think it could be doing her any good.

Then came Session 4. The instructor was leading a meditation practice that began with focusing on the breath and then expanded the field of awareness around the breath to include a sense of the body as a whole. At first Maria was not aware of any body sensations. Then she registered a sense of something unpleasant, a slight sensation around the top of her stomach, just below the ribcage in the middle of her body. It was not strong, nor painful, but it was there: a sort of empty feeling, a slight stretching at the edges, unpleasant to focus on, but interesting in that she had never noticed it before. As she held this bundle of sensations in awareness, she was aware of the image of her son and daughter, then an image of their empty rooms in the house. The sensations passed, and for the first time in her life she left that session feeling more intrigued by an unpleasant feeling state than afraid of it.

Now, a few days later, and in her empty house after the children had left, she emptied the wastepaper basket and went upstairs to put it back. Once again, she felt a wave of sadness. But this time, rather than chasing it away, she allowed herself to sit on the edge of the bed and tune in to wherever these feelings were affecting her body. She became aware of the feeling just below the ribcage and felt a tiredness in her arms and legs. She held all these sensations in awareness and for the first time was able to get a sense of space around them, as if air was moving around, under, and over the sensations. She started to cry but did not try to stop it. She felt lonely but did not try to deny it to herself. She felt angry with herself and her husband but did not feel that it was wrong to feel this way. She found that she was sobbing but did not feel either out of control or in control—the issue of control seemed irrelevant. It must have been one or two minutes later when the crying changed; there were moments of quiet, and a stillness; then some more tears, and then again, the stillness. Somehow she felt at peace, although nothing had changed. And she wasn't afraid anymore. She got up, put the wastepaper basket in the corner of the room, and went to get ready to go to work.

For Maria, the practice of widening attention around the breath to include a sense of her whole body offered a way to move beyond her habitual avoidance to a willingness to experience what was on her mind and what she was carrying in her body. There are many different ways in which we can reconnect with ignored or pushed away aspects of ourselves. By sampling a range of mindfulness practices over time, we can ultimately each find our own unique way back to befriending and learning from our full range of emotions. In that spirit, let's look at two more practices that might help us be more mindful and more accepting of our sometimes elusive feelings. The first uses a diary sheet to help us tune in to pleasant and unpleasant moments as we go about our day; the second can be used to further explore the feel of things—learning to read our own body sensations as if it were a "physical barometer."

Awareness of Pleasant and Unpleasant Moments

Making a commitment to be aware of pleasant or unpleasant feelings in any moment requires that we be sensitive to what is actually going on for us inwardly. Of course, this requires *tuning in, the exact opposite of experiential avoidance.* Forming the explicit intention to be aware of what is pleasant or unpleasant in a particular experience and how it feels in the body, in the heart, and in the mind can not only help us to become more aware of the

> ### BECOMING AWARE OF THE PLEASANT AND UNPLEASANT QUALITIES OF EXPERIENCE
>
> How can we become more aware of feelings (pleasant, unpleasant, or neutral) and of the physical sensations in our bodies in our daily lives? You might like to try this:
>
> Over the next few hours, be on the lookout for even the smallest moments when you register an experience as "pleasant" or "unpleasant." You can use the Pleasant and Unpleasant Event Calendars on pages 232–233 and 235–236 to keep a record of what was actually going on in the moment in question, with particular attention to the interplay of feelings, thoughts, and physical sensations during each event. Recording what you were actually experiencing in each instance can be very valuable.

actuality of our experience, but also begin to reverse the automatic habit of experiential avoidance.

This was exactly Sam's experience when, as part of the mindfulness course in which he was participating, he had spent a week looking out for pleasant moments in his everyday life. His experiential avoidance had been so extreme that he often found himself falling asleep when he was not busying himself with one thing or another, or scrolling on his phone, even though he was not actually physically tired. It seemed that sleep—or scrolling— provided him with a way to numb out from the world of feeling. In the early sessions of the program, Sam came across as somewhat withdrawn and disengaged. Then came Session 3. There seemed to be a change in Sam: he looked animated and engaged; he smiled. When participants were invited to report back on their experience with the Pleasant Events Calendar, Sam described how he had discovered that his life was far richer in pleasant events than he had imagined: the smile of a passing acquaintance, the reflections of trees on water. Without making any changes to the actual pattern of his day, Sam had discovered many small sources of happiness that were already there in his life, waiting to be found. All he needed to do was to deliberately tune his attention to what had always been available to him. This availability was revealed only when he deliberately focused on the world around him and was more prepared to experience feelings. Naturally, he was happy; but that was not the main point of the exercise. What Sam was exploring was how to take the risk of engaging with moment-to-moment living as it actually was, rather than tuning out of it for fear of what it might become.

> We can cultivate awareness of feelings from different angles: pay attention to the moment and see what sensations arise, or notice a particular pleasant or unpleasant feeling and pay attention to the thoughts, other feelings, and sensations that are present along with it.

Reading Our Own Barometer

There is a second practice that can help to bring awareness of feelings into our everyday lives—it's called the "Body Barometer" and was developed by

Trish Bartley. The instructions can be found on the facing page. By first directing attention to a general area of the body (such as the torso) and then asking us to identify a particular pattern of subtle bodily sensations within that general area (a combination of physical body sensations and the intuitive feelings of pleasantness/unpleasantness/neutrality), these instructions allow us to discover what is often a previously unsuspected resource. For many, this resource has provided very helpful guidance and enrichment for everyday life.

We have touched on a number of reasons we might choose to put time and effort into cultivating a wider and deeper awareness of our bodily experience: it connects us with the here and now; it reduces experiential avoidance and enables us to connect more fully with life; it allows us to process body sensations and feelings less automatically; it disrupts the vicious cycles that fuel unhappiness and bias our thoughts and judgments.

The point of recognizing when situations evoke unpleasant feelings, or

---

THE BRIGHT FIELD

I have seen the sun break through
to illuminate a small field
for a while, and gone my way
and forgotten it. But that was the pearl
of great price, the one field that had
the treasure in it. I realize now
that I must give all that I have
to possess it. Life is not hurrying

on to a receding future, nor hankering after
an imagined past. It is the turning
aside like Moses to the miracle
of the lit bush, to a brightness
that seemed as transitory as your youth
once, but is the eternity that awaits you.

—R. S. THOMAS, *Collected Poems*

THE BODY BAROMETER

If you have an old-fashioned barometer or have seen one, you will know that you use it by gently tapping on the glass front. Depending on which way the needle moves, it is possible to forecast upcoming weather. We can use our bodies in a similar way to give us sensitive information about upcoming emotional "weather."

Here is how you do this:

1. Determine some part of the body—preferably in the trunk—such as the chest area or the abdomen or somewhere between the two—that for you is especially sensitive to sensations of stress and difficulty. You can put your hand there.

2. Once you have found the place, it can become your "Body Barometer." Tuning in to it regularly, you will notice different sensations at different times. When you are under pressure, feeling anxious, or irritable, you may notice sensations of tension, tightness, shakiness, or discomfort. The intensity of these sensations varies, depending on the level of your difficulty.

3. As you practice this, you can become aware of quite subtle sensations. These may signal that something is just beginning to emerge, long before you are aware of this in the mind. If you wish, you can practice coming to the breath, or do a Breathing Space (see Chapter 9) to help you turn toward and gently "hold" what is happening. Or you may choose just to monitor the sensations in your "barometer," moment by moment, and be with them as they are.

It takes only a few moments to turn to the Body Barometer to discover what is there. Like so many of the short mindfulness practices, it's easy to practice. The challenge with them all is to remember. How will you remember to check in to your Body Barometer? Can you set up a reminder specifically for this? If you can practice this a few times every day for a couple weeks, you will establish it as a resource readily available to you.

when our contracted bodies tell us we have already reacted with aversion, is that we can then learn how to *respond* more skillfully. Can we learn how to *be with* an unpleasant feeling in a way that is not going to get us trapped in obsessive preoccupation, endless cycles of rumination, and thus persistent unhappiness and depression? Can we transform our very relationship to our emotions? It is to this possibility that we turn in the next chapter.

Seven

Befriending Our Feelings

How could we forget those ancient myths that stand at the beginning of all races, the myths about dragons that at the last moment are transformed into princesses? Perhaps all the dragons in our lives are only princesses who are only waiting to see us act, just once, with beauty and courage. Perhaps everything that frightens us is, in its deepest essence, something helpless that wants our love.

So you must not be frightened if a sadness rises in front of you, larger than any you've ever seen; if an anxiety, like light and cloud shadows, moves over your hands and over everything you do. You must realize that something has happened to you, that life has not forgotten you, that it holds you in its hands and will not let you fall. Why do you want to shut out of your life any uneasiness, any misery, any depression, since after all, you don't know what work these conditions are doing inside you?

—RAINER MARIA RILKE, *Letters to a Young Poet*

Anyone who starts out on an adventure knows that there will be obstacles along the way that may seem insurmountable. Climbers train for months, knowing that gentle slopes will give way to large overhangs that look impossible to scale. Trail runners pore over detailed maps and will walk or run the route several times until they can see in their sleep the terrain they'll cover on the day of a race. Still, no amount of preparation entirely eliminates the challenge of the real thing. We have now reached just such a critical juncture in our quest to reverse the cycle of unhappiness.

The challenge before us at this point is to see if we can be with our unwanted emotions without making them worse. The very notion may seem strange and the task impossible because we so easily fall into aversion and the driven-doing mode. Yet such an intentional, conscious gesture, which amounts to a paradoxical embrace of what we fear most, can be a powerfully liberating act. Yes, the mind's readiness to leap in to meet difficult emotions in problem-solving mode, its aversion to unpleasant experiences, and our reflexive self-castigating response to even fleeting sadness may all stand in our way. But mountain climbers reach "impossible" heights all the time by *using the skills and knowledge they have developed in the course of their training.* Working through this book offers training in exactly the skills and the knowledge needed right now to address the challenge of our most difficult emotional states.

In the last chapter, we explored a group of exercises that can help us tune in to the body's signals of aversion and unpleasantness. We may have gotten so adept at avoiding negative emotions in the past that we no longer recognize them or the aversion that would serve as our "getaway car." In this chapter, we'll go one step further and learn to *recognize, approach, accept,* and *befriend* those emotions so that they do not so easily trigger a downward spiral into depression.

Befriending emotions that we've viewed as the "enemy" for so long may run counter to all of our self-preservation instincts. But, when it comes right down to it, what else is there to do? The alternative so far has been to struggle and suffer whenever things have not gone as we had hoped they would. Perhaps it's time to explore another path.

We are not claiming that cultivating mindfulness in the face of a tendency toward sadness, low mood, and depressive rumination is easy. But it *is* doable. What is more, it draws on what is deepest and best in us. In this book we offer many suggestions for relating more skillfully to unpleasant experience. But ultimately, through the cultivation of mindfulness, each of us will discover *our own ways* to transform our relationship with what we find unpleasant, difficult, and threatening.

Making use of the mindfulness practices we have already described, we are well on the way to reversing our habitual rejection of the difficult and the unpleasant. Bringing a gentle openness and interest to something troublesome is, in itself, an enormously important part of acceptance. It will be invaluable if we can remind ourselves, again and again, of a simple but powerful truth: *intentionally holding something in awareness is already an affirmation that it can be faced, named, and worked with.* In fact, it is also an immediate embodiment of facing it, naming it, and working with it.

Placing Our Trust in Body Awareness

The key here is to uncouple our experience of unpleasant feelings from the knee-jerk reaction of aversion that habitually follows it—or, if we are already caught up in aversion, to free ourselves from its grip. Just as we were able to focus on body sensations to help us identify aversive reactions, we can work mainly through the body to respond more effectively to the events that trigger aversion. Working through the body keeps difficulties in play long enough for us to discover that even the worst circumstances we find ourselves in are indeed workable. This is particularly crucial to keep in mind when every fiber of our instinctual being is telling us to fix or get rid of the difficulty as quickly as possible.

Whenever something unpleasant arises, the systems in the brain that warn us about potential threats are activated: it is as if a loud alarm is sounded, and the mind gives high priority to attending to whatever caused the unpleasantness. We may do many things to try to distract ourselves—such as doomscrolling through social media—but the alarm is insistent and doesn't shut off. Worries keep intruding on our consciousness. Sooner or later, with our phones in our hands or not, the disturbing thoughts and feelings come flooding back.

Here is that critical moment. If, paradoxically, we can turn and *face* whatever it is that we are finding scary, difficult, or depressing rather than perpetually distracting ourselves to no avail, we are actually still doing what the brain wants us to do: giving high-priority attention to the matter at hand. It's just that we are no longer giving it attention in the old "doing" way. We are approaching the moment—whatever it is and however it is— not by *reacting* but rather by *responding*, by bringing *an open, spacious, and affectionate attention* to the feeling in the moment *as it expresses itself in the body.* Now we are in relationship to the alarm in a new way, one that provides us with a viable alternative to endlessly *thinking about* it.

By now we have seen time and again how we react automatically to difficult emotions by triggering the driven-doing mode, so dominated by thinking. The sequence may begin with our worrying about all the things that could go wrong and would make things worse, and then move on to what to do about it. We dig up old memories and get caught in the stream of endless rumination. Because these reactions all register as "unpleasant" on our internal barometer, another unconscious cycle of aversion is triggered.

But now there is another possibility. The very fact that we are learning to read this internal barometer and can be aware of this attempt to push away the unpleasant, and that we can locate the accompanying uncomfortable sensations *in the body*—as muscle tightening and overall contracting, or bracing—gives us the opportunity to use this information from the body to break the downward spiral into rumination and depression. *We do this by trusting ourselves to hold difficult feeling states in awareness—an awareness that includes how they feel in the body.* By opening up even the tiniest bit of breathing room—between the experience of "unpleasant" when first detected and the tendency to react almost instantaneously with aversion—we give ourselves powerful and precious opportunities to nourish and shape our ability to see and *respond* to what is happening. We tap into the deep wisdom in our own mind, a wisdom that does not rely on thought, to respond to difficulties in ways that can be transformative and freeing. Here's how:

Once we notice an unpleasant feeling, we focus, as best we can, on *how we experience it in the body.* This is aided enormously by connecting our awareness of the breath in that very moment with whatever the unpleasant experience is—what we were calling in Chapter 6 the gesture of "breathing with." This breathing with whatever arises in and of itself tends to steady the mind. As discussed in Chapter 6 (pages 129–130), it involves expanding the awareness of our breath sensations to include awareness of other relevant sensations we are experiencing in the body. Practicing in this way includes intentionally *breathing in* to any area of painful or uncomfortable sensations, exploring its "edges" and any changes in intensity, and allowing our awareness to simply hold it all. In such a moment, we have an opportunity to recognize any signs of aversion manifested in the body as contraction. Tying awareness of the breath to awareness of other sensations in the body makes the breath a vehicle for the movement of awareness just as it was in the body scan. But since this awareness can also hold thoughts and feelings, if those should arise, the field of awareness can readily recognize and accommodate them as well, without having to do anything at all. The awareness itself does all the work.

We can start to learn this new way to relate to unpleasant sensations and feelings through the mindful yoga introduced in the last chapter. You may like to read the following section and then put the book down for a few minutes and do some of these stretches, following along with audio guidance on Track 3 (*www.guilford.com/williams3-materials*). As best you can, approach these stretches in the spirit we now describe.

Working the Edge

We almost inevitably encounter at least some degree of bodily discomfort in key places when we practice stretching through mindful yoga. This is what makes this practice such an effective vehicle for learning how to approach difficult and unwanted moments and experiences with greater acceptance, curiosity, gentleness, and kindness. What is more, the new skills we develop in working with even a mild degree of physical discomfort can be directly applied later to situations of emotional discomfort, however intense they may be.

Let's imagine we have our hands above our heads, we are stretching upward with our whole bodies, and it is beginning to feel uncomfortable in our shoulders and upper arms. One way to react (the *avoidance option*) is to back off as soon as we feel any discomfort, perhaps immediately lowering our arms and turning our attention to some other part of the body or even out of the body altogether, maybe into a stream of thoughts or images. Another possibility (the *unkind option*) is to grit our teeth, tell ourselves we just have to put up with the increasing pain and discomfort, and not make a fuss, as if this were the aim of the practice. We would then put even more effort into pushing ourselves to stretch further. Here, too, we are likely to numb out, removing our awareness from those regions of the body experiencing the discomfort.

But there is also a third option, one that strikes a balance between withdrawing at the first sign of discomfort and forcing ourselves to meet some self-designated standard of endurance. This *mindful option* calls for approaching the situation in a spirit of gentle nurturing, using the stretch to extend our ways of relating to discomfort. We direct our attention right into the area of discomfort as best we can, using the breath as a vehicle to bring awareness right into that region, as in the body scan. With a gentle curiosity we then explore what we find there—physical sensations and feelings, coming, going, and changing. We sense them directly, perhaps focusing on any changes in intensity over time. The idea is not to hold a posture until it is painful. It is rather to experience the limit of the movement in any particular stretch or posture and then to linger there without forcing or pushing through strong sensations. All the while we keep our attention on the sensations and feelings themselves, as best we can. We focus on the physical qualities of the sensations, on any sense of tightness, holding, burning, trembling, or shaking, *breathing with* the sensations, as best we can. We allow our thoughts about what these feelings mean to simply come and go in awareness.

We can play with the intensity of sensation by actually varying the stretch itself, experimenting with working the edge of our discomfort and our acceptance, exploring for ourselves just how the body responds directly to every tiny change we introduce. This approach gives us some sense of being able to modulate the intensity of unpleasant sensations. This is also a way we can be gentle and nurturing toward ourselves while still learning how to relate to whatever arises in a new way. We don't try to force things beyond our limit of the moment.

The body provides a wonderful arena in which we can directly witness the effects of aversion and the power of an accepting awareness to dissolve it. For example, as we continue to hold our arms stretched out above our heads and we become aware of an increasing sense of discomfort, we might invite ourselves to briefly scan the body to see if we can pick up regions where the muscles are tense and contracted, even though they are not directly involved in holding up the arms. It is quite common to become aware of tension and contraction in the face, such as the jaw or forehead. Clearly, these regions are making no essential contribution to holding the arms up. Why, then, are they contracted? Their contraction is simply a sign that we are reacting with aversion to the experience of discomfort. Knowing this, we can breathe a gentle, curious, nurturing attention into these regions of the body on the in-breath while on the out-breath we allow ourselves to let go of any sense of resistance or holding. As best we can, we let any tension leave with the out-breath, to the extent that it will. In all likelihood, a sense of increased ease and lightness in the face will give us direct feedback that we have mindfully released ourselves, to one degree or another, from our automatic habit of tensing and bracing in aversion against discomfort.

> The face can be a "weather vane" for the tension that signals aversion in action. Increased softness in the muscles of the face can indicate some degree of mindful release from aversion.

Mindful stretching provides a very useful training ground for exploring new counterintuitive ways to respond to discomfort. It also offers, in itself, an invaluable way to shift modes of mind when we feel ourselves sliding into unhappiness. We can put on audio Track 3 (www.guilford.com/williams3-materials), for instance, and perhaps recover our clarity of mind just by attending to the body's movements and sensations over a relatively short period of time. When our mood has deteriorated, when we may be finding it difficult to concentrate, it is helpful to be able to ground ourselves in awareness of the tangible sensations that arise as we stretch and twist and work with our bodies. This gentle yet always challenging physical activity can also have a direct enlivening and arousing effect that may cut through the lethargy that can rear its head as unhappiness deepens. In fact, it is very difficult to remain sad or anxious while doing yoga in a mindful way. It is as if we were literally and metaphorically sweeping the body clean—and, along with it, the mind.

WORKING THE EDGE IN SITTING MEDITATION

We described in Chapter 6 (pages 129–130) how we might run into a certain degree of discomfort in the sitting meditation simply by being still for an extended period of time, even more so when sitting cross-legged on the floor. One or both knees, the back, neck, or shoulders might start to ache, and the ache can intensify with time, sometimes quite dramatically. Recall that the sitting meditation invites us to first let our attention settle on the breath sensations themselves, and then gradually expand the field of awareness once it is relatively stable, to include a sense of the body as a whole or any particular regions that might be giving rise to intense sensations.

So here is another effective opportunity, just as in the mindful yoga, to develop our ability to work the edge, befriending our experience in the body by turning toward and opening to whatever is present, even if our initial reaction is strong aversion. As we saw in Chapter 6, when our attention is repeatedly drawn to such uncomfortable sensations, we can include those areas of greatest intensity within the field of awareness and experience them moment by moment just as they are, even if it is just for a few moments at first. Here we are again, working the edge, gently and lovingly zeroing in on our boundaries and limits by moving into and embracing the sensations themselves, until we sense that we have reached our limit for the moment. Then we intentionally and caringly back off, and shift our attention from the region of greatest intensity, ready to return when we have gathered and regrouped our resources. We might do this in a number of ways:

■ One possibility is to shift attention within the general region of intensity; rather than focusing on the region of maximum intensity, we focus on an area of lesser intensity.

■ Another possibility is to *breathe with* the discomfort, holding awareness of the intense sensations together with awareness of the breath, in the background.

■ Or, if the intensity is becoming overwhelming, we can shift the focus of attention away from that region entirely and focus attention exclusively on the breath.

■ And we always have the option of moving the body intentionally, of shifting our posture during the sitting meditation practice if the intensity becomes too great. This is an act of kindness and intelligence in itself and not a measure of failure. And we can be aware of shifting our posture too, so that there is a continuity of awareness regardless of how we are responding to the intensity of sensation.

The point here is that the practice itself allows us to discover different ways to stay in relationship to our inner experience, even when it is unpleasant and difficult. It reminds us that we don't have to throw ourselves in all at once. It's more like dipping just the big toe in the water to test the temperature.

What we are learning here about the power of awareness to contain whatever arises without our needing to push it away or to try to escape from it, can be applied to any other intense experience of physical or emotional pain. We discover that we can take care of ourselves by actually embracing and befriending *whatever* we are feeling in awareness, an awareness suffused with qualities of kindness and a gentle openness and interest in what is arising within us—*whatever* it is.

> **With the shift from trying to ignore or eliminate physical discomfort to paying attention with friendly curiosity, we can transform our experience.**

ANTHONY'S STORY

Anthony's experience illustrates the transformation that cultivating mindfulness makes possible. He had come to mindfulness classes because he felt constantly tense and ill at ease. Yet focusing on his body had simply made him more aware of his discomfort. He could not just "be with" the feelings of tension in his body at first. He kept wanting things to be different and was frustrated that he did not feel any better when he tried to meditate. Then one day while walking in the woods his dog disturbed a hornets' nest. After dragging his dog away, Anthony found his own leg covered in the insects. Several stung him, and he had to get home quickly to put on some ointment. After a day or two, the stings had stopped being painful but had become intensely itchy. Anthony had been told emphatically not to scratch, but he could hardly bear it, so strong was the itch. He decided to experiment with bringing his awareness to the itching and discomfort, "breathing into it" to investigate it more closely. He noticed that the itching was not just one sensation but many. What's more, this bundle of sensations changed from moment to moment, some of the sensations shifting rapidly, some more slowly.

Later, Anthony was able to apply the skills he had developed in dealing with the physical discomfort of itching to discomfort related more directly to emotion. When his body felt tense, rather than getting fed up or trying to ignore it, he was now able to stay inside the tension, breathing with it, moving up close to it, in intimate contact with the various sensations associated with it. He found that he was able to bring a greater sense of compassion toward his body and a more accepting attitude toward himself.

Anthony was learning the difference between avoiding (shutting him-self off from experience) and approaching (being open to experience) the difficult. He discovered that the difference can be very subtle, yet very liber-ating. Such a sense of freedom comes because the shift from avoidance to openness is accompanied by a shift from the brain pattern that underlies avoidance to a new brain pattern that underlies approach. As in the mouse-in-the-maze experiment this new pattern allows for a greater flexibility of response.

> For now, we are building trust in the body and our ability to take care of ourselves.

When we are able to sense in the body that we are tensing up or bracing ourselves in anticipation of something threatening, that is an indicator that the brain is switching into *avoidance* mode. In response, our mindfulness brings in *approach* qualities such as curiosity, compassion, and goodwill, and balances out the brain's tendency to switch into its *avoidance* pattern with a pattern associated with "welcoming."

Mindful awareness and learning to be with unpleasant feelings are not about striving for some ideal of happiness in the face of the difficult—that would be just another goal we are fixating on. Rather, it is as if we are bath-ing the difficult situation, and even our aversion to it, in an open, compas-sionate, and accepting awareness, just like a parent embracing a suffering child. We can take this stance not only toward *physical* discomfort but also toward *emotional* discomfort.

Approaching Difficult Emotions

Unpleasant emotions are invariably accompanied by sensations and feelings in the body. If we gently focus our attention *right into* these areas of intense sensation and discomfort, we bring about both immediate and longer-term effects. We immediately short-circuit any unhelpful avoidance tendencies of the mind. We also disrupt the automatic links among body sensations, feelings, and thoughts that perpetuate vicious cycles and downward mood spirals. In the longer run, we develop more skillful ways of being in rela-tionship to uncomfortable experiences. Rather than seeing them as "bad and threatening things," a view that triggers avoidance and gets us stuck in suffering, we begin to see unpleasant experiences for what they are: passing mental events—bundles of bodily sensations, feelings, and thoughts. As best we can, we greet them with a sense of interest and curiosity, rather than with a sense of unease, hatred, and dread. We welcome them in, as they are already here anyway.

In the MBCT program, we have specifically designed a practice for investigating the texture of emotionally challenging situations. The practice helps us explore and cultivate more skillful responses in those critical moments by deliberately inviting a difficult scenario or circumstance to come to mind. We then work with it in the body, bringing awareness to it, breathing into it, and discovering a wider space within which it might exist. The instructions follow (pages 150–151), and you'll find audio guidance on Track 10 at *www.guilford.com/williams3-materials*, narrated by Mark Williams.

AMANDA'S STORY

Amanda, a participant in our program, had trouble with this practice at first. When asked to bring a difficult situation to mind, her first reaction was "I'm not sure I'm going to be able to do this. I can't think of anything." She got worried that she was going to miss out on this exercise. Then suddenly something came into her mind. It had to do with her son.

"He's been giving us a really hard time recently—staying out all hours, hanging around with people we don't trust. We had a real crisis two months ago involving the police. As soon as this came into my mind I knew this was going to be difficult to get out of my mind again. I try not to think about it at all, but every time I do, I think *Where have I gone wrong?*"

Amanda believes she won't be able to get this difficulty out of her mind because her experience is that she has "failed" at it before. She is now judging and blaming herself, questioning what she has done to produce this dilemma. Notice that this troubling situation immediately sets off the driven mode of thinking that we call "rumination."

The next instruction, to focus on body sensations and feelings, was very difficult for her. Initially it was as though her breathing had stopped completely. Then she recognized that large areas of her body were extremely tense. Normally, she would have tried desperately to think of something else—to distract herself, to think positively. But here she was being invited

INVITING A DIFFICULTY IN AND WORKING WITH IT THROUGH THE BODY

Track 10 of the audio files at *www.guilford.com/williams3-materials*

Preparation

1. Sit for a few minutes, focusing on the sensations of breathing, then widening the awareness to take in the body as a whole.

Bringing a Difficulty to Mind

2. When you are ready, see if you can bring to mind a difficulty that is going on in your life at the moment, something you don't mind staying with for a short while. It does not have to be very important or critical, but it should be something that you are aware of as somewhat unpleasant, something unresolved. Perhaps a misunderstanding or an argument, a situation where you feel somewhat angry, regretful, or guilty over something that has happened. If nothing comes to mind, perhaps you might choose something from the past, either recent or distant, that once caused unpleasantness.

Tuning In to the Physical Sensations

3. Now, once you are focusing on some troubling thought or situation—some worry or intense feeling—allow yourself to take some time to tune in to any physical sensations in the body that the difficulty evokes. See if you are able to note, approach, and investigate inwardly what feelings are arising in your body, becoming mindful of those physical sensations, deliberately directing your focus of attention to the region of the body where the sensations are strongest in the gesture of an embrace, a welcoming. This gesture might include breathing into that part of the body on the in-breath and breathing out from that region on the out-breath, exploring the sensations, watching their intensity shift up and down from one moment to the next.

4. Once your attention has settled on the bodily sensations and they are vividly present in the field of awareness, unpleasant as they may be, you might try deepening the attitude of acceptance and openness to whatever sensations you are experiencing by saying to yourself from time to time: "It's okay for me to feel this; whatever it is, it's already here." Then just stay with the awareness of these bodily sensations and your relationship to them, breathing with them, accepting them, letting them be, allowing them to be just as they are. It may be helpful to repeat "It's here right now. Whatever it is, it's already here. Let me open to it." Soften and open to the sensations you become aware of, letting go of any tensing and bracing. Say to yourself "softening" or "opening" on each out-breath. Remember that by saying "It's okay to feel this," you are not judging the original situation or saying that everything's fine, but simply helping your awareness, right now, to remain open to the sensations in the body. If you like, you can also experiment with holding in awareness both the sensations in the body and the feeling of the breath moving in and out, as you breathe with the sensations moment by moment.

5. And when you notice that the bodily sensations are no longer pulling your attention to the same degree, simply return 100 percent to the breath and continue with that as the primary object of attention.

6. If in the next few minutes no powerful bodily sensations arise, feel free to try this exercise with any bodily sensations you notice, even if they have no particular emotional charge.

Ending

7. As the practice comes to an end, bring your attention back to the sensations of the breath, or to the body as a whole as you sit for a few moments.

to bring attention to, and to breathe into, those regions in her body that felt most tense. Realizing just how tense she was in that moment, Amanda purposefully expanded her attention to include the whole body and breathed into the places where the tension and contraction were most intense.

Then something totally unexpected happened. She suddenly became aware that she could give those feelings some room. "It suddenly became like a great big empty space, with the air coming in and out," she said. "You know, sometimes when you come back from a vacation and the house is a bit musty, so you open all the doors and windows to let the air blow through? Well, it was like that—having doors and windows open, with curtains blowing and air coming in and out. And it was really amazing. The tension about my son was still there. I thought, *Oh, you're still there, but never mind—the wind's blowing through, and that's all right.*"

The unexpected difference seemed to be that Amanda could look at the difficulty. The feeling in her body was still a bit tight, but the area of tension seemed to be much smaller, with a sense that the air could flow around it.

Amanda's experience shows that it is indeed possible to work with difficult feelings and memories in a way that acknowledges them, allows them to exist, and does not push them away. We can so easily think of meditation as a clever way to *get rid* of these frightening states of mind. But it is important to keep in mind that mindfulness is not about getting rid of anything, nor is it about "not having" such feelings arise in the first place. Rather, the intention behind cultivating mindfulness of emotional states is to learn how we can relate to them in ways that will not get us stuck in unhappiness. One way of knowing that we are on the right track is having a sense of spaciousness in how we are holding these feelings. The feelings are still here, in this very moment, just as they were for Amanda, but it is as if, somehow, they do not take up all the space in the mind. They are seen and held in a greater awareness, an awareness that is discerning and openhearted. And, interestingly enough—and this is something you can explore for yourself and play with—the awareness *itself* is not in pain, or unhappy, or caught in any way at all.

Amanda's description of her experience with her particular difficulty is revealing. "To begin with," she said, "it was like a solid mass of rock. It was huge. It was so solid that you couldn't get around it, but then it shrank to a small stone. It was still stone, but it was small. It's really good. Because I think probably I have been pushing the issue away, sort of sitting on it and not letting it come up fully to the surface. I haven't allowed it before to simply be here. I thought it would just overwhelm me. It was too much to let in, and so my natural reaction would have been just to tense up and push it away and not face it at all."

> Deliberately bringing attention to the difficult with the hope that this will help to get rid of it may simply get us more stuck.

Amanda was discovering the transformative power of allowing something to be here as it is. As with the mouse-in-the-maze experiment described in Chapter 6 (pages 122–123), the same action performed to escape from a feared object can have very different consequences than when it is motivated by approaching the positive.

MEG'S STORY

The point of the practice we have just described is to provide, within the laboratory of a therapeutic program and the meditation practice itself, opportunity after opportunity to explore and develop more effective ways of responding to unpleasant feelings and emotions. These skills, developed in this admittedly highly contained formal learning situation, can then be used where they are really needed: in our everyday lives. Sometimes the effects can be quite dramatic, as Meg found out:

"I awoke yesterday feeling really angry. I was fuming. I knew exactly what it was about. The day before I had had a meeting with my supervisor (I was doing an evening course to get qualified and we've all got to do a project). She had promised to read my draft project write-up before we met so she could give me feedback on it. The deadline is coming up soon, and I had lots of other work to do, so I needed her comments now so I could work on it over the holiday. When I got there, she apologized and said she hadn't been able to get to it yet. She'd been away, et cetera, et cetera. She flicked through it and gave me some general comments for how to redraft it and said I'd be fine. The meeting finished, and I felt pretty much okay about it. I decided to start redrafting it the next morning and went to bed. That was the day before yesterday.

"But the morning after I'd seen her, I woke up really bitter. I had all these angry thoughts going round and round in my head: *She knew when the draft was arriving; she just doesn't care. Perhaps she doesn't want to supervise me. Well, if that's how she feels, I'll leave the course. I don't have to continue. I'll simply leave a note for her and tell her I'm not coming back to the class. She'll be sorry then.* I told myself that I was stupid to be thinking like this, that I was overreacting. But as soon as I thought I had calmed down, another angry thought would come, or I would imagine her opening my note or imagine me walking out of college.

"I suppose I lay there for about five minutes, fuming away. Then I remembered something we had learned about what to do when we get locked into this sort of self-talk: about moving away from thinking—and shifting awareness to how the thoughts and emotions were felt in my body. I shifted my attention to my body and was able to feel, very clearly, a tightness in my chest and stomach. I lay in bed and simply held in awareness the sense of these feelings as they were occurring in my body. The next moment the sensations were gone and with them the anger. Just like that, in a flash. I couldn't believe it; like a soap bubble I had just touched—and it disappeared.

"I got up, went over to my desk, turned on my computer, and worked on redrafting the project. Although from time to time since, I still think of her not reading the work, it does not have the same ability to charge me up."

This almost looks like magic. Indeed, people who have been through mindfulness-based training programs sometimes use words such as *miracle* to describe experiences like Meg's. As mindfulness develops, we can more and more observe thoughts and emotions as if they were bubbles rising from the bottom of a pot of boiling water; we simply watch as they burst at the surface. It sometimes feels as if the awareness itself, in touching the thought or feeling, makes it go "poof," just like Meg's soap bubble. Teachers in the Tibetan tradition sometimes say in this regard that thoughts "self-liberate" in the field of pure awareness.

Meg's experience shows that, when we experience difficult and unwanted emotions, we can transform our experience by intentionally bringing a kindly/allowing awareness to these feelings and emotions as they are experienced in the body. Once more, we see that cultivating awareness by working through the body in the very moments that the first inklings of emotional reactivity arise allows us to sidestep a possible descent into persistent unhappiness and depression. It provides a way to be with any persisting unpleasant feelings without struggle, offering the possibility of fully experiencing being alive, even in the midst of whatever difficulties we are challenged with.

Taking the Path of Honesty and Openness

By now it should be clear that working with difficulty through the body does not mean just grimly thinking about its awfulness. Mindfulness is hardly an exercise in either stoicism or thinking. Anthony, Amanda, and Meg had the courage to bring full awareness, coupled with elements of curiosity and self-compassion, to their experience. As a result, their relationship to their difficult emotions shifted dramatically.

In the past, the tensions that they each felt in their bodies were associated with trying to protect themselves from being overwhelmed by such difficult feelings. But all that did was to freeze the normal unfolding and resolution of an emotional process. Aversion and avoidance, and all the tension that surrounds them, prevent us from moving beyond old wounds and old habits of self-criticism.

Gaining the basic confidence to let down our habitual and instinctive defenses unconditionally in the face of difficulty is certainly bound to take some time. Sometimes, particularly in those who have survived severe trauma, doing this kind of work effectively requires a protected and highly supportive therapeutic environment. Each of us needs to choose a pace at which we can work the edge of painful and difficult feelings, especially if they involve painful memories.

This attitude of radical acceptance is expressed simply and profoundly in the poem "The Guest House" by Rumi, a 13th-century Sufi poet.

Turning toward such feelings and being willing to experience them is a very brave thing to do, but it can also seem like a crazy thing to do since it

---

THE GUEST HOUSE

This being human is a guest house.
Every morning a new arrival.

A joy, a depression, a meanness,
some momentary awareness comes
as an unexpected visitor.

Welcome and entertain them all!
Even if they're a crowd of sorrows,
who violently sweep your house
empty of its furniture,
still, treat each guest honorably.
He may be clearing you out
for some new delight.

The dark thought, the shame, the malice,
meet them at the door laughing,
and invite them in.

Be grateful for whoever comes,
because each has been sent
as a guide from beyond.

—RUMI, *The Essential Rumi*

runs counter to all our commonsense instincts for self-preservation. In the final analysis, however, if we want freedom from the habitual reactivity of the mind, we may have no choice—in the end, the path of honesty and genuine openness may be the only path that offers healing and resolution. The alternatives may just not go deep enough or may suffer from lack of authenticity.

The beauty of bringing a wider moment-by-moment awareness to an old wound, a current pain, or a difficulty is that it opens up new possibilities for our minds and our bodies. It's saying: "Let's come to this afresh. Let's allow the difficulty to be here—I'll just be with it now, in each moment, as if it were a sick child in the middle of the night that needs to be held tenderly and reassured."

> Radical acceptance can keep us from becoming progressively constricted and diminished in the face of painful experiences. It invites us to fully experience the richness of life even when things seem to be at their worst.

In mindfulness practice, a spirit of gentleness and tenderness is combined with a spirit of adventure and discovery: "Let's see what is in this moment . . . and this moment . . . and this moment." This means that we've got only the problems of this moment—and they may not even be a problem in *this* very moment—rather than piling on all the problems of next week, next year, and the rest of our lives, which we so reflexively fall into doing. If our thoughts persuade us that our lives will always be like this ("*This is just how I am*"), then what started with pain or tension or sadness is going to give rise to even greater suffering. But if we're just here *for* this moment, and *in* this moment, with *these* thoughts and feelings and body sensations, and now in the very next moment the mind's patterns are changed in some way, and now, changed again in the very next moment, events have a chance to unfold in an entirely different way. And yet it is always now, and therefore always "workable" in the very same way as "The Guest House" is suggesting.

THE WISDOM TO BE GAINED FROM BEING WITH DIFFICULT EMOTIONS

Suspending judgments and shifting our perception of difficult emotions can help us enormously. Unpleasant emotions are an ever-changing constellation of physical sensations, thoughts, and feelings, just as pleasant ones are.

They seem to have a life of their own, but they can be met and embraced in awareness. Coming to terms with our emotions means seeing deeply into them. At the heart of healing, and of the healing gesture we make toward ourselves, is gentle, kind acceptance of whatever we find right in the midst of the difficulty itself. These discoveries can be surprising. We might find that fear keeps rising to the surface of our awareness even when we are not conscious of being afraid of anything in particular. We might notice, for the first time, a deep aching emptiness. Perhaps we'll find that a dull ache that seems to be with us all the time in fact ebbs and flows, rises and falls, and is composed of a variety of feelings that we would not describe as an ache at all. Just knowing and radically accepting that these feelings are part of us in this moment can help keep the mind from turning on the "aversion switch" that leads to desperate brooding over how to get rid of the feelings.

A focus on the sheer physicality of difficult experiences can catalyze this important shift in perception. It can also help us become familiar with our own specific, distinctive pattern of bodily sensations that signal aversion. Learning to recognize these patterns helps us identify them more quickly. Then, seeing that characteristic pattern as it pops up time after time in our lives can powerfully support the view of difficult emotions as neither a problem nor a threat . . . and aversion itself as simply an old habit. Eventually, we may even recognize it simply as a very familiar and frequent visitor: "Oh, here you are again." By witnessing, over and over again, the effects this visitor has on us, we may begin to see ever more clearly that such visitations do no good at all for us or for anyone else and also that they are nowhere near as powerful as we sometimes think, in spite of all the misery they can carry with them. This realization can help ease us out of the grip in which aversion can hold us.

It also affects our experience of suffering. Whether you will still be in pain after you begin to practice mindful awareness is

> **Avoiding the difficult is a compelling old habit. But there is an alternative.**

impossible to say. We can know a moment only when it arrives, only when we look into it. What we *can* say is that if there is pain and it can be held with the sense of openness that Rumi invokes, it will be more bearable than otherwise. There may still be pain, but there also may be less suffering.

By bringing mindful awareness to what is actually unfolding in our experience, we're not necessarily going to change the rock-bottom sensations in the body. But there is every chance that we will see what's going on with greater accuracy and precision. And that gives us the power of choice. We can *decide* to be in an entirely different relationship to old mental habits. We can decide either to open to all the sad or angry thoughts and feelings with awareness, as suggested in "The Guest House," or to succumb to our habitual tendency to withdraw and turn away.

Our old habits may try to persuade us that avoiding the difficult is necessary. But this is not true. There *is* an alternative. We can free ourselves from the things that hold us down and hold us back. Once we know how to look, we will see that our world holds much more promise than we might have imagined from inside the prison of our discontent.

Eight

Seeing Thoughts
as Creations of the Mind

Imagine you are twelve years old and in school. The day is dragging, but you brighten up when you remember that it's Wednesday. Your dad has promised to pick you up after school to take you to buy new running shoes. It's been seven months since your mom and dad split up. You miss your dad, and so you look forward to these shopping trips.

After school, you don't wait for the bus with the other kids. You stay in the school building for a while and then wander out toward the road. Your dad's not there, but that's okay. He'll have been held up. He never misses. Ten, then fifteen, minutes go by, and you see some of your teachers in their cars leaving the school. One of them stops to ask if you're okay, and you say "Fine." Half an hour later, it's starting to get dark. All the school buses have long since left.

You start to worry about where your dad is. Has he had an accident? Has he forgotten you? Surely not. You've tried calling but his phone is switched off. You've left a text but he hasn't replied. You remember other times you've felt alone. You start to feel miserable. You wonder where everything went wrong. School hasn't been good; you don't really have a good friend like the other kids.

You try to cheer yourself up. What's on TV tonight? It doesn't work. Your favorite program was yesterday, Monday evening. Monday? That means today isn't Wednesday! You got the day wrong. You feel silly, but also relieved, happy even. You run back into the school and ask the janitor if you can call your mom.

How did you feel as you read through the scene and imagined yourself as that child? What went through your mind?

You may have noticed, imagining yourself as the child, that your feelings depended first on what you were thinking and imagining about what had happened to your dad at each stage, and second on what that brought to mind about things generally in your life. In this scenario it's easy to see how some thoughts, activated by one event, bring to mind other thoughts and feelings. For example, feeling lonely because he has been left by his dad leads the child to thoughts of not having as many close friends as others—for many of us, this is a feeling that persists into adulthood.

The turning point of the story occurs when the child realizes that he has mixed up the days. This new piece of information, that it isn't Wednesday, completely changes how the child sees the situation. Changes in emotion follow the change in perspective.

Although this is only a story, we can all recall situations in which we have misinterpreted things, just as the child in the story did. It is often only on these sorts of occasions that we see how much our emotions depend on our *interpretation* of situations. Most of the time we don't get such a reality check.

We are always explaining the world to ourselves, and we react emotionally to these explanations rather than to the facts.

There is nothing particularly mysterious in the way the mind is working here. The mind creates a narrative, a story to fit the facts as we see them. And once created, the story may be very difficult to dismantle. Yet that story can have alarmingly powerful effects on our emotions and feelings. It can press our emotional buttons, even if it is a complete or partial fiction with little basis in reality. All the feelings experienced by the child—the worry about his father, his sense of abandonment, his feeling of loneliness—were brought about by an event that never actually happened. The child only *thought* his dad was failing to turn up at the promised time.

A century ago, Sigmund Freud popularized the idea that we all have an unconscious that lies deep below the surface of our awareness, motivating our actions in ways that are highly complex and that take considerable time to unearth and understand. Those in mainstream academic psychology rejected such ideas as unprovable and focused instead on observable behavior (in a movement known as "behaviorism"). So fierce was this reaction against Freud that it was only in the late 1960s and the 1970s that behaviorally oriented psychotherapists started to take seriously the interior world of their patients: the subjective domain of thoughts, memories, ideas, predictions, and plans. And they made a remarkable discovery: most of what drives our emotions and behavior is not deeply unconscious, but just below the surface of our awareness. Not only that, but this rich interior world, with its motivations, expectations, interpretations, and storylines, is accessible to all of us if we dare to look. We can all become more aware of the "stream of consciousness" going on in our minds, moment by moment. It often takes the form of a running commentary. If it is potentially damaging to us, it is not because it is buried deep in the psyche but because it is virtually unattended. We have gotten so used to its whisperings that we don't even notice it is here. And so, it shapes our lives.

Once we have reacted to a particular situation, we rarely go back to check on whether our interpretation was actually accurate. Of course, it is entirely possible that a father might have really forgotten to pick up his child. It does happen. But most often our minds do not consider a range of options; our first impressions, reactive as they are, are usually taken as an accurate readout on reality—the way it *really* is.

The self-narratives we construct soon get set in concrete as reference points for the future—regardless of how far they are from representing the truth of the here and now.

The example of the waiting schoolchild and of the scenario in Chapter 1—in which you were asked to imagine a friend failing to acknowledge you from across the street—show how even small differences in our mood and thinking can determine our whole perspective on an event. These little shifts in mood and thought end up entangling the mind, creating more feelings and downward mood spirals as the thinking mind ruminates on and on to find answers that don't come. And so we create a story—a "drama about me"—that may gradually wander far away from the here and now and far away from the way things actually are. Once the script we have concocted for ourselves has been set in the mind, we may unwittingly rely on it as a reference point for all present and future judgments—without ever checking back with the here and now. Without knowing it, our thoughts become words carved in stone rather than words written on water.

Seeing Thoughts as Thoughts

As we saw in Chapters 1 and 2, our thoughts influence our feelings and body sensations and are themselves influenced by our feelings and body sensations. But that does not make our thoughts true, no matter how compelling they may feel.

As we have seen, in mindfulness-based programs one very effective strategy for regaining mental balance is to attend to the direct experience of feelings in the body. As far as thoughts themselves are concerned, through mindfulness we can cultivate a new and very different *relationship* to them, allowing thoughts simply to be here instead of analyzing them, trying to work out where they came from, or trying to get rid of them in any way. In awareness, we see them immediately for what they actually are: constructions, mysterious creations of the mind, mental events that may or may not accurately reflect reality. We come to realize that our thoughts are not facts. Nor are they really "mine" or "me."

> The realization that thoughts are not facts is vitally relevant to all of us.

When cultivating mindfulness, we adopt this orientation because if we can perceive a thought such as "I'm always going to feel this way" *as* a thought, we instantly rob it of its power to upset us. It can no longer force us to go round and round trying to avert a feared (yet totally imaginary) situation. Mindfulness practice invites us to see more clearly the link between thoughts and feelings. But our task is not only to become *more* aware of our thoughts, but to become aware of them *in a different* way, to relate to them from within the being mode of mind. In being mode, it becomes much clearer which thoughts are helpful and which are merely the endless "propaganda" of depression.

If you have been practicing the meditations described up to this point, chances are that your relationship with your thoughts has already begun to shift. Maybe you occasionally find yourself responding differently (perhaps even smiling) when you catch yourself jumping to the "usual" doom-and-gloom conclusions or assumptions: "She's trying to undermine me and make me look foolish," "I'll never get this job done," "I always say the dumbest things." Maybe you don't start to brood as quickly following such thoughts. Or perhaps you've begun to notice that something that used to trigger immediate upset can now come to mind without you getting charged up by it—you can just let the thought, with all its potential baggage, float by.

Such changes may reflect the fact that, perhaps without realizing it, you have already begun to learn how to respond more skillfully to your thoughts *during* meditation. The act of registering in awareness that the mind is wandering involves a shift from being totally absorbed in a thought stream to being detached enough from it to see what has happened. And each time we gently label our thoughts as "thinking" and intentionally disengage from the thought stream, we reinforce the shift in relationship toward seeing thoughts *as* thoughts. They are mental events that pass through the mind like clouds or weather patterns pass through the sky.

HEARING OUR THOUGHTS

A thought arises, lingers in consciousness for a relatively short while, then fades. It's just a mental event, an "object" that we can pay attention to but that is neither "me" nor reality. But sometimes we may need a more concrete way to shift our perspective so as to perceive it in that way. Our sense of hearing may provide such a way.

Sounds are around us all the time. We don't need to go out and hunt them down. We can just give ourselves over to hearing what is already here to be heard in this very moment. Sounds are just part of the input the mind receives from the world.

These facts determine how we normally relate to sounds. When we hear the sound of a truck in the street, we don't automatically think of it as part of ourselves; we know it is on the street outside.

> **Think of it this way: the mind is to thoughts as the ear is to sounds.**

If we think of the mind as the "ear" for our thoughts, then perhaps we can learn to relate to thoughts that arise in the mind in the same way that we relate to sounds arriving at the ears. Normally we may not even be aware of the extent to which the mind is "receiving" thoughts until we refine our ability to be aware of them, until we practice intentionally giving them the space to simply be here as they are and to be seen and known for what they are: discrete events in the field of awareness. By analogy, mindfulness of *hearing* can help us develop a similar sense of openness toward our thoughts, allowing them simply to come and go, without enticing us into the drama they are creating.

In the practice on pages 165–166, we attend to sounds (mindfulness of hearing) for a time and then move to seeing if we are able to relate to thoughts and thinking in the same way. In this way, we are creating optimal conditions to remain with that way of attending to experience while we shift the focus of our attention from sounds to thoughts. You can follow the instructions for this practice of mindfulness of hearing and thinking on audio Track 6 at *www.guilford.com/williams3-materials*.

CARRIED AWAY BY THE THOUGHT STREAM

Just as the mind will wander during other meditation practices, from time to time most of us will find that our mind has been drawn into a particular thought stream and carried away during the preceding exercise. Returning to the movie metaphor, it's as if the mind has left its seat and gotten sucked into the action up there on the screen, now playing a part in the story that it was mindfully observing the moment before. When we realize that this is happening, all we need to do is acknowledge that the mind had been caught up in the thought stream and that now awareness has been reestablished. It is helpful to notice any emotional reaction or intensity arising from any element of the storyline and then, gently and compassionately, to escort the mind back to its seat, back to observing the play of thoughts and feelings. If at any time we feel our mind has become unfocused and scattered, or if it repeatedly gets drawn into the drama of our thinking and imagining, it is always possible to come back to the sensations of the breath in the body, using the breath as an anchor to gently steady and stabilize our attention.

> At least to begin with, we suggest you focus your attention specifically on thinking for no more than five minutes at a time.

It is important to acknowledge the difficulty of this practice; we are so used to living inside our thoughts rather than attending *to* them that it can be extraordinarily challenging to maintain a mindful relationship to thinking for any length of time.

We must be careful when working with thoughts in this way. There is a fine line between taking a friendly interest in our thoughts as mental events

MINDFULNESS OF HEARING AND THINKING

Track 6 of the audio files at *www.guilford.com/williams3-materials*

Preparation

1. Practice mindfulness of breath and body as described in the instructions for Mindfulness of the Breath and Body in Chapter 6 (Track 5), until you feel reasonably settled.

Awareness of Hearing

2. When you are ready, allow the focus of your awareness to shift from sensations in the body to hearing—bring your attention to the ears and then allow the awareness to open and expand so that there is a receptiveness to sounds as they arise, wherever they arise.

3. There is no need to go searching for sounds or listening for particular sounds. Instead, as best you can, simply open your mind so that it is receptive to awareness of sounds from all directions as they arise—sounds that are close, sounds that are far, sounds that are in front, behind, to the side, above, or below—opening to the whole space of sound around you. Allow awareness to include obvious sounds and more subtle sounds. Allow it to include the space between sounds and silence itself.

4. As best you can, be aware of sounds simply as sounds, as bare auditory sensations. When you find that you are thinking *about* the sounds, reconnect, as best you can, with direct awareness of their sensory qualities (patterns of pitch, timbre, loudness, and duration), rather than their meanings or implications.

5. Whenever you notice that your awareness is no longer featuring sounds in the present moment, gently acknowledge where your mind has drifted off to, and then return your attention back to hearing sounds as they arise and pass away moment by moment.

Awareness of Thoughts as Mental Events

6. When you are ready, let go of featuring sounds and instead feature thoughts center stage in your awareness. Just as you were aware of whatever sounds arose—noticing their arising, lingering, and passing away—so now, as best you can, allowing your awareness to discern any and all thoughts that may arise in the mind in just the same way—noticing thoughts arise, as they linger in the space of the mind, and as they eventually dissolve and disappear. There is no need to try to make thoughts come or go—just let them come and go on their own, in the same way that you related to the arising and passing away of sounds.

7. You might find it helpful to bring awareness to thoughts in the mind in the same way that you would if the thoughts were projected on the screen at the movies—you sit, watching the screen, waiting for a thought or image to arise. When it does, you attend to it as long as it is there "on the screen," and then you let it go as it passes away. Alternatively, you might find it helpful to see thoughts as clouds moving across a vast spacious sky. Sometimes they are dark and stormy, sometimes they are light and fluffy. Sometimes they fill the entire sky. Sometimes they clear out completely, leaving the sky cloudless.

8. If any thoughts bring with them intense feelings or emotions, pleasant or unpleasant, as best you can, note their "emotional charge" and intensity and let them be as they already are.

9. If at any time you feel that your mind has become unfocused and scattered, or it keeps getting repeatedly drawn into the drama of your thinking and imaginings, see if it is possible to come back to the breath and a sense of the body as a whole sitting and breathing and use this focus to anchor and stabilize your awareness.

and becoming seduced by their content and emotional charge. We can be virtually bushwhacked and bamboozled by them, drawn imperceptibly into believing that they are true and they are us and we are them. Once we "become" them, we can slide down the well-greased grooves of the doing mode and fall back all too easily into ruminative brooding. This new relationship to thoughts may not be too difficult to hold for brief periods of time. But, in the earlier stages of practice, the longer we attend to our thoughts, the more likely we will be drawn into them and mesmerized so that we lose our mindful perspective on them.

Meditation teacher Joseph Goldstein puts it neatly:

When we lose ourselves in thought, identification is strong. Thought sweeps our mind and carries it away, and, in a very short time, we can be carried far indeed. We hop a train of association, not knowing that we have hopped on, and certainly not knowing the destination. Somewhere down the line, we may wake up and realize that we have been thinking, that we have been taken for a ride. And when we step down from the train, it may be in a very different mental environment from where we jumped aboard.

If we find ourselves taken hostage and carried away by the thought stream, it makes sense to steady and gather the mind (Chapter 4) by focusing on the breath and remembering that every in-breath is a new beginning and every out-breath a release, a new letting go.

Noticing Self-Critical Commentary

Although we may practice with thoughts as our primary focus of attention for only a few minutes at a time, there are innumerable other opportunities to apply and extend this new perspective. The more we engage in the various formal meditation practices, the more we may notice ourselves having reactions to what we are experiencing, judging how well things are going, and criticizing ourselves if we think we're not feeling what we are "supposed to be" feeling or that we are "not very good" at meditating. Such moments can be hard to capture, as such judgmental thoughts—like many thoughts about ourselves—seem to creep into the mind "under the radar." Yet they are wonderful opportunities to remember that judging and criticizing are really just more thinking. Can we, at such times, relate to these patterns of thinking as mental events? It can help to recall how we relate to the less charged thoughts and images during the formal practice of mindfulness of thoughts. Practicing in this way allows us to bring this relationship to thoughts into more and more of our moments, freeing ourselves from their grip and allowing our inherent wisdom to discern their wider movements and patterns within the mind. With time, we may come to experience an open, spacious quality in our awareness that easily holds whatever is arising in the domain of mind or body (including any judgmental thoughts) and learn to rest in that awareness itself.

Jacob found that his daily meditation practice was frequently accompanied by a running critical commentary: *You've lost it again. Can't you even stay focused on your breath for half a minute at a time? This is a waste of time. You're messing this up just like everything else you try. Can't you get anything right? What's wrong with you? What a failure you are!* At first he found this commentary an upsetting, albeit familiar, "interference" obstructing and undermining his attempts to get on with "the proper business" of meditation, which he saw as keeping his attention firmly focused on the breath. This is a common experience. Gradually we may come to realize that awareness of these patterns of thought *as* thoughts *is* meditation. How can we help ourselves to see this?

GIVING NEGATIVE THOUGHT PATTERNS A NAME

One possibility is to give a name to the patterns of thinking that habitually occur. We can use labels such as "Judging Mind" or "Hopeless Mind" or identify them as subpersonalities: "My worst critic," and so on. The important thing is that we have a way of pointing to the common threads and general themes that cut across a range of specific contents in our minds. Ideally, the labels that we choose should help us drop into a wider and wiser perspective on these thought patterns. Such labels may help us see them, with some degree of nonattachment, as frequent visitors to the mind rather than identifying with them as parts of ourselves or hearing them as the voice of truth or reality.

Jacob found that he could label the whole critical, judgmental package as "Critical Mind." Once he had done that, he was able to look out for the visits of Critical Mind and greet it as an old, if not wholly welcome, acquaintance. This enabled him to let Critical Mind come and go without giving it the power to trigger the cascade of negative thoughts that would normally have quickly mired him in the negativity with which he was already so familiar.

NEGATIVE THOUGHTS IN THE LANDSCAPE OF DEPRESSION

Identifying negative judgmental thoughts as recurring mental patterns can be of enormous help in allowing us to relate to them more objectively and less personally. Those of us who have experienced depression in the past can take this process a step further if we can see negative thoughts for what they often are: well-known features of the landscape of depression. They are not reliable readouts on truth or reality.

Are any of the thoughts in the exercise below familiar to you, from your own experience? If you've experienced periods of depression in the past, seeing this list may take you back, not wholly willingly, to the thoughts that dominated your mind at those times. Even if you haven't experienced

RECOGNIZING AUTOMATIC NEGATIVE THOUGHTS

The following is the same list of automatic thoughts reported by people who were currently depressed that we saw in Chapter 1.

As you look at the thoughts in the list, think about how strongly, if at all, you would believe each of the thoughts if it popped into your head *right now*. If you choose, you could assign each one a number from 0 to 10 to indicate the strength of belief.

1. I feel like I'm up against the world.
2. I'm no good.
3. Why can't I ever succeed?
4. No one understands me.
5. I've let people down.
6. I don't think I can go on.
7. I wish I were a better person.
8. I'm so weak.
9. My life's not going the way I want it to.
10. I'm so disappointed in myself.
11. Nothing feels good anymore.
12. I can't stand this anymore.
13. I can't get started.
14. What's wrong with me?
15. I wish I were somewhere else.
16. I can't get things together.
17. I hate myself.
18. I'm worthless.
19. I wish I could just disappear.
20. What's the matter with me?
21. I'm a loser.
22. My life is a mess.
23. I'm a failure.
24. I'll never make it.
25. I feel so helpless.
26. Something has to change.
27. There must be something wrong with me.
28. My future is bleak.
29. It's just not worth it.
30. I can't finish anything.

When you have finished, think back to a time when you were at your most depressed and then return once more to the list. Think now about how strongly you would have believed each of those thoughts had they occurred *at that time*.

prolonged bouts of depression, you may recall having thoughts similar to these when feeling "down."

Jade, when asked during our program whether any of the thoughts on the list were familiar, said, "Yes—all of them." For her this exercise revealed a crucial distinction: "When I was in the middle of the depression, I believed the thoughts 120 percent—this was how things were, no question—I was just 'seeing the truth,' grim though that seemed. But now—now that I'm feeling okay most of the time—I don't often have these thoughts, and if I do they just seem to be faint echoes of how they were then. Looking back, I just wonder how I could ever have believed all that stuff. *I'll never make it*—yes, that's just how it seemed, there was absolutely no hope of getting through the depression—and yet here I am!—living proof that I did."

This simple exercise has some profound implications. When we are depressed and experience these thoughts, they don't feel like just thoughts. They seem to be telling the truth about us, our self-worth, and the state of our lives. But almost everyone who experiences depression has very similar thoughts. That suggests a very different possibility: these thoughts are part of the territory, the landscape, of depression. They are symptoms of depression in just the same way as aches and pains are symptoms of the flu. When we have the flu, our temperature goes up and down. We may alternate between saying "It's too cold in here" and getting a blanket and "It's too hot in here" and opening a window. Our temperature is being created by the virus, not the temperature in the room. So it is with negative thinking. The intensity of negative thinking is created by our depressed mood, yet we take the thoughts to be real—to be revealing the truth of things.

Negative, self-critical thoughts come and go as part of depression. Viewed in this way, these thoughts are informative, but not in the way we might have imagined. They tell us a great deal about the thinking patterns that go along with depression, about the way a low mood can affect our thought processes. They tell us very little about the real state of ourselves or the world or the future.

> **Negative thoughts are part of the landscape of depression. There is nothing personal about them.**

This alternative way of viewing such negative thoughts comes across particularly powerfully when people go through a mindfulness-based cognitive therapy program with others who, like them, have experienced multiple episodes of depression but are now relatively well. When they all answer "Yes—all of them" or something similar to the question about their familiarity with the automatic thoughts, something remarkable happens. A moment of realization that "This is depression—it's not me" seems to occur for many. The class participants view one another as "normal" people—friendly, supportive, funny. Every last one of them has at some point, in the depths of despair, harbored the private conviction that "It's me—only me—who is no good." Now they realize that other people have the same negative automatic thoughts while depressed—and believe them with every fiber of their being. Suddenly they don't feel quite so alone. More than that, they begin to see how powerful depression is: how terrifyingly persuasive it can be. When we were at our worst point, we were *convinced* that we were the world's worst person and that the future was doomed, and now, perhaps only a few weeks later, we look back and wonder, incredulously, *How could I ever have thought that?*

> **Our thinking will often reflect our mood and our mode of mind, not what is "actually" here or who we actually are. Thoughts are not facts.**

If we can adopt the perspective of allowing thoughts to be seen and known and recognized in awareness for what they are, in *this* moment, our relationship to them will be altered in the *next* moment. In that way, we can free ourselves from their entangling, distorting, harming potential.

Jade had always assumed that only by analyzing her thoughts ("spiraling off into analyzing," she called it) could she reduce their destructive effects. Then, during one practice period, she suddenly realized, "All this analysis that I try to do—it isn't making it *less* scary, thinking about it like that. It's making it *more* scary!"

Through mindfulness meditation practice, Jade was catching a glimpse of the possibility of the freedom that comes when we are able to let go of identifying with our thoughts, the freedom that comes from resting in awareness, watching thoughts come and go like clouds (or even storms) in the mind. She caught a glimmering of the power of not taking things so personally when, in actuality, they were impersonal events and hardly reliable

> Intellectualizing and analyzing doesn't work when low mood has been triggered. Remembering that thoughts are "just thoughts" is a wiser strategy.

carriers of absolute truth. With this insight Jade found she was released from having to analyze everything. She saw that thinking things through too easily got her lost in an endless labyrinth of memories and worries.

"Actually, simply staying with all of this might be less frightening than analyzing it," she said. "That's a totally new idea for me: staying with it may be healthier than analyzing it."

Befriending Thoughts *and* Feelings

It's incredibly valuable to recognize automatic negative thoughts, among other thinking patterns. Tuning in to them and seeing them for what they are gives us another opportunity to disrupt the depression cycle—to break the chain from a different angle. Still, these thoughts are usually just the tip of the iceberg. The tip can be valuable in alerting us to the larger mass below. But if we wish to reduce the threat from the iceberg as a whole, it may not be particularly effective to focus exclusively on the tip. If we dynamite the tip away, a new section of iceberg will simply rise above the surface, and if we wish to navigate safely around the iceberg, we would do well to assess the scale of the submerged portion rather than adjust our steering to avoid only what we can see.

Although our thoughts obviously affect our feelings, the thoughts themselves originate in underlying, less perceptible feelings: the base of the iceberg. Those feelings may persist just on the edge of awareness long after the individual negative thoughts "born" of them have arisen, passed through the mind, and disappeared. So it's usually helpful, once we acknowledge the presence of thoughts as mental events, to go underneath the thought level and work through directly sensed body experience—the feelings we get from an unpleasant experience (such as a sense of anger) as well as physical sensations (such as tightening in the shoulders). To do this, we bring an affectionate and discerning awareness to each aspect of our felt emotions, as best we can, using the meditation practices from Chapter 7. We may notice changes from moment to moment—for example, the transformation of a sense of anger to a sense of hurt, then to a softer sense of sadness. We will revisit working in this way in Chapter 9 and Chapter 10.

The exploration of the ecology of our thoughts and feelings is particularly difficult when our thoughts are about a painful past event or about current unfinished business that seems to call for immediate action. Then the thoughts seem to have real power over us. An effective response is not to ignore them but to see them clearly, with awareness. When we let them come and go, we remain free to choose which thoughts are appropriate, even wise and healthy; which to listen to, believe, and possibly act on; and which to simply recognize as unhelpful and let pass.

> **Seeing clearly that our thoughts are mental events is particularly difficult when they are related to a painful event in the past or when the mind tells us they are high-priority unfinished business.**

In doing this work, we are learning how important it is to bring mindfulness to those times that we become alerted to the presence of unpleasant thoughts and feelings. It is tempting at such times to instantly switch our attention away as soon as we detect that the thoughts or feelings are unpleasant and to return our focus of attention back to the haven of the breath. But it is more skillful to pause long enough to bring to them a spirit of gentle inquiry and curiosity, an investigative awareness: *Ah, there you are; let me see who you are.* In this way, we not only develop a new perspective toward them, seeing them, increasingly, as passing events in the mind. We are also in much better shape to become familiar with the *content*

> The key to awakening from the bonds of fear is to move from our mental stories into immediate contact with the sensations of fear—squeezing, pressing, burning, trembling. . . . In fact, the story—as long as we remain awake and don't get stuck in it—can become a useful gateway to the raw fear itself. While the mind will continue to generate thoughts about what we fear, we can recognize the thoughts for what they are and drop under them again and again to connect with the feelings in our body.
>
> —TARA BRACH, *Radical Acceptance*

of recurring messages. Furthermore, this sense of openness, curiosity, and exploration will activate the approach mode of the mind and brain. In itself, this will directly counteract the avoidance mode and so provide a further steadying influence that can prevent us from getting caught up in and carried away in all our own imaginings.

Identifying and naming our recurrent thought patterns is one way to help us see the virtual "audio or video tracks" in the mind for what they are. Recognizing them when they are starting up allows us to say: "Ah, I know this track; this is my 'I'm a total failure' track or my 'I'll never be happy' track." This will not necessarily switch it off, or if it appears to, it will almost certainly return soon. The difference will be in the way we relate to it: as a fact that we can do little about, or as a highly conditioned and inaccurate "track" running in the mind that will continue to be an inconvenience until it ceases of its own accord.

Amazingly, in the domain of the mind, this cessation can come about naturally, without any forcing or struggling, when we are able to see, to grasp, to understand what is going on with clarity and self-acceptance. We gradually see that it is natural not to like what is unpleasant and so allow the unpleasantness to be felt without the need to push it away or fight with it—"It's okay not to like this." In this understanding is the release and the cessation. This is the cardinal characteristic of awareness and clear seeing. It is embodied and inhabited through the gift of mindfulness practice, a gift we can give to ourselves over and over again. Yes, it involves a good deal of discipline, but that discipline itself, the willingness to look and actually to see, is in fact a truly valuable gift we can give ourselves.

Beyond Thoughts and Feelings: Choiceless Awareness

Up to this point, we have described the practices of mindfulness meditation as they are taught sequentially in the mindfulness program, one after another: mindfulness of taste; mindfulness of the movements of the breath; mindfulness of body sensations lying down, as we stretch, move, and walk; mindfulness of pleasant, unpleasant, and neutral feelings; mindfulness of aversion; mindfulness of sounds; and finally mindfulness of thoughts and emotions. Each of these practices directs us repeatedly to focus our attention in a specific way on a particular aspect of our experience. In this way, we are progressively cultivating our capacity to be mindful, to develop the skills that can free us from unhappiness and depression.

All the various practices that we have visited so far cultivate awareness in relation to particular objects of attention. All of them illuminate different aspects of our lives and of our interior landscapes. But these divisions are somewhat arbitrary; the awareness we have been cultivating is the same whether it remains focused on the breath, on tasting, on bodily sensations, or on feelings or thoughts.

The next practice unifies all these separate strands of training in mindfulness and reveals them to actually be elements of one seamless whole. This is the practice of choiceless awareness (see page 176). This is the final extended formal practice we will introduce. In the next chapter, we consider how our developing mindfulness skills might be carried from formal and protected settings to the more challenging informal practice settings of everyday life. This is where our need for them is most urgent and where they can be most useful.

To begin cultivating choiceless awareness in formal practice, we can include a few minutes of it at the end of any of the other practices we are engaged in, as is the case toward the end of Track 6 and Track 11 of the audio guidance (www.guilford.com/williams3-materials). It's always possible to jump to choiceless awareness at any moment, simply by letting go of any and all objects of attention. This sounds easy, but it is in fact a very challenging practice because we have nothing specific to focus on. We rest in open awareness itself, without any attempt to direct our attention toward anything other than awareness itself. There is no need even to think that you are meditating or that there is even a "you" to meditate. Even these are seen and known as thoughts by awareness, and in the seeing, in the knowing, they are seen to dissipate, again, like touching soap bubbles.

As we engage in this practice, we may become increasingly aware of the distinction between the objects to which we can direct our attention, if we choose, and the space of awareness in which all our experiences arise. The objects could be thought of as celestial bodies hanging in space. In choiceless awareness, we become the space that holds whatever condenses momentarily within it. Awareness, like space, is boundless, having no edges

CHOICELESS AWARENESS

In the early stages of this practice, it might be wise just to play with it for relatively short periods of time, returning to the breath or featuring some other specific chosen object of attention at other times. It sounds so simple to "just sit" without any chosen object to attend to—to simply be awareness itself, to be the knowing. It is not so easy. Yet with time and motivation, the practice of choiceless "open" awareness can become more and more robust and more and more compelling.

We begin with a few minutes of focusing on the breath (Track 4), and then, if we care to, we allow the field of awareness to expand to include any or all of the following: body sensations (including the breath; Track 5), sounds, thoughts, and feelings (Track 6).

Then, whenever we feel ready to, we see if it is possible to let go of any particular object of attention, like the breath, or class of objects of attention, like sounds or thoughts, and let the field of awareness be open to whatever arises in the landscape of the mind and the body and the world. We simply rest in awareness itself, effortlessly apprehending whatever arises from moment to moment. That might include the breath, sensations from the body, sounds, thoughts, or feelings. As best we can, we just sit, completely awake, not holding on to anything, not looking for anything, having no agenda whatsoever other than embodied wakefulness.

This practice invites us to be completely open and receptive to whatever comes into the field of awareness, like an empty mirror, simply reflecting whatever comes before it, expecting nothing and clinging to nothing; awareness itself attending to the entire field of present-moment experience in utter stillness.

There is audio guidance that includes breath, body, sounds, thoughts, and choiceless awareness at Track 11, narrated by John Teasdale.

or limits. The invitation is to settle into this awareness, to *be* the knowing, the nonconceptual knowing that pure awareness actually is. Awareness is not itself subject to pain, although it bears profound and empathic witness to pain. And so once we have become acquainted with it, we may find it easier simply to hold even the most difficult and painful of our experiences within it. We may even make the curious, but profound, discovery that awareness is already free, intrinsically whole, and deeply knowing.

Nine

Mindfulness in Everyday Life

TAKING A BREATHING SPACE

> Mindfulness is neither difficult nor complex; *remembering*
> to be mindful is the great challenge.
> —CHRISTINA FELDMAN

Those of us who attempt to nurture greater mindfulness in our lives sooner or later discover that it is most difficult to be mindful at just those times when mindfulness would be most helpful. When the pressure is on, when we're feeling bad, when there doesn't seem to be a moment to spare, these are the times when being mindful can be a major challenge. They are also the times when we need it most.

Mindfulness is at least as much about ordinary daily living as it is about making some quiet time for formal practice. In fact, we could say that ultimately life itself is the practice; there is no waking moment in which we might not be more alive and more in touch if we were more aware. So the real work of mindfulness actually starts with life itself, with all its twists and turns, in all its guises and disguises. This is especially so when life is particularly difficult, when it is hard going, when the mind is all over the place. At such times we most need the stability, the clarity, and the insight that mindfulness offers. In this chapter, we gather together the threads of all we've learned so far to see how we can weave our discoveries into the fabric of our daily lives.

From the outset, both the mindfulness-based stress reduction (MBSR) program and the mindfulness-based cognitive therapy (MBCT) program emphasize the importance of bringing mindfulness to everyday life. They invite us to pay attention to routine activities such as brushing our teeth, feeding a pet, or taking out the garbage (Chapter 3); to walk mindfully when we are walking (Chapter 4); to use sensations in our bodies as a way to stay aware and present in each moment (Chapter 5); and to support mindfulness of any experience by "breathing with" it (Chapter 6). The MBCT program also offers a special tool that is specifically designed to bring mindfulness into our everyday lives, particularly at the tipping points when our mood is beginning to go down. The tool is a mini-meditation called the three-minute breathing space. In MBCT it is always used as the first step in dealing with difficult situations and feelings.

> The three-minute breathing space is used as the first step in responding to whatever challenging situations and feelings arise in a particular moment.

In the breathing space, the entire teaching of the MBCT program is concentrated in three steps. Many of those who have participated in the program have singled this practice out as the most useful feature of the whole course. When so many of our daily tasks seem to require doing mode's critical thinking, this practice offers a quick and surprisingly effective way to switch to being mode when we most need to do so.

One way to experiment with this would be to start by reading the instructions on the facing page all the way through, then diving in and taking a three-minute breathing space right now. Alternatively, you could follow the instructions on audio Track 7 at *www.guilford.com/williams3-materials*. You may find it helpful to spend about a minute on each of the three steps, or you might want to vary the times (for example, by spending somewhat longer on Step 2).

At first we practice this breathing space for three minutes at set times, three times a day, in a rather formal way. But once we have the hang of it, it can be deployed anytime, anywhere, for the duration of one or two breaths, to five to ten minutes, as conditions permit. Soon we may find we are using it, to some degree or another, in many situations, such as when we notice unpleasant feelings or a sense of "tightening" or "holding" in the body or feelings of being overwhelmed by events. In such situations, when low mood threatens to overwhelm us, the breathing space allows us to see clearly what is happening through direct, experiential knowing. It allows us to steady ourselves. It provides a place from which we can choose mindfully what responses are required by the situation we find ourselves in.

THE THREE-MINUTE BREATHING SPACE

Track 7 of the audio files at *www.guilford.com/williams3-materials*

Preparation

Begin by deliberately adopting an erect and dignified posture, whether you are sitting or standing. If possible, close your eyes.

Step 1. Becoming Aware

Bringing your awareness to your inner experience, ask: What is my experience *right now?*

- What *thoughts* are going through the mind? As best you can, acknowledging thoughts as mental events, perhaps putting them into words.
- What *feelings* are here? Turning toward any sense of emotional discomfort or unpleasant feelings, acknowledging their presence.
- What *body sensations* are here right now? Perhaps quickly scanning the body to pick up any sensations of tightness or bracing.

Step 2. Gathering

Then redirect your attention to focus on the physical sensations of the breath breathing itself.

Move in close to the sense of the breath in the belly . . . feeling the sensations of the belly wall expanding as the breath comes in . . . and falling back as the breath goes out.

Follow the breath all the way in and all the way out, using the breathing to anchor yourself in the present.

Step 3. Expanding

Now expand the field of your awareness around your breathing so that, in addition to the sensations of the breath, it includes a sense of the body as a whole, your posture, and facial expression.

If you become aware of any sensations of discomfort, tension, or resistance, zero in on them by breathing into them on each in-breath and breathing out from them on each out-breath as you soften and open. If you want to, you might say to yourself on the out-breath,

"It's okay for me to feel this; whatever it is, it's already here"

As best you can, bring this expanded awareness into the next moments of your day.

In the first step of the breathing space, having stepped out of automatic pilot, out of doing mode, we are asked to come fully into the present moment. We intentionally suspend our usual habits of self-critical judgment; we let go of trying to get somewhere other than where we already are. We practice restraining our usual tendency to fix what the doing mind thinks needs fixing. We simply acknowledge and bring awareness to what is already here in this moment, as it is.

Sustaining this open stance of acknowledging and attending can be very difficult. Old habits of thinking have well-worn grooves that can easily carry us away. So we take the second step, of gathering and focusing our mind on a single object: the sensations of breathing, just this breath coming in, just this breath going out. In this way, we give ourselves a chance to steady the mind and to remain right here, right now. And if for any reason the breath is not a stable enough anchor for our attention (which can happen in those who suffer from asthma, panic disorder, or COVID symptoms), we can gather our attention by focusing on the sensations in the feet or hands or the contact that our body is making with whatever is supporting it at that moment.

Having gathered ourselves by focusing attention in this way, we take the third step. We expand the field of awareness to include the whole body. We enter the spaciousness of the being mode and, as best we can, allow that wider domain of being to be with us when we return to what we were doing. These three steps help us shift seamlessly from the mode of doing to the mode of being.

For most of us, bringing mindfulness into the busyness of everyday life may turn out to present a big challenge. The breathing space was developed to allow *a deliberate change of stance toward what is going on*, in any moment. In a potentially difficult situation, this shift in mode may be essential for an effective and appropriate response. For this reason, the three-minute breathing space is more structured and directive than many of the other practices described so far. In particular, we start with a definite change in posture, and we remind ourselves that there are three different stages to the practice (for example, by using the phrases "Step 1," "Step 2," and "Step 3"). The use of such an explicitly structured approach to the instructions is not accidental. The shorter a practice, the more likely the tendency for it to become merely a brief time-out, snatched in the midst of an ongoing crisis, rather than a major shift in our mode of mind—from driven-doing to being.

It might help to think of the path that our attention travels in the breathing space as having the shape of an hourglass. An hourglass has a wide opening, a narrow neck, and a wide base. This image can remind us to open to experience as it is in Step 1, to gather attention to focus on the breath or other anchor in Step 2, and to open to a sense of the body as a whole in Step 3.

> **Think of your attention during the breathing space as traveling a path with the shape of an hourglass.**

The breathing space needs to have the qualities of a sharp and discerning sword; used with compassion, it can cut through the doing mode to provide us with a powerful and healing alternative. The practice can open up new freedom and choice about how best to respond to what is happening in our lives, inwardly and outwardly while it is happening.

The breathing space forges an explicit link between the formal practices described in the preceding chapters and daily life. It picks up the threads of the learning that naturally unfolds during regular formal practice and weaves them into the fabric of everyday life. The breathing space's Step 2, "Gathering," is like a concentrated version of Mindfulness of the Breath (Chapter 4). Step 3, "Expanding," resonates with the formal practices of widening the attention around the breath to include a sense of the body as a whole (Chapter 6) and embracing a difficulty (Chapter 7). The significance of Step 1 may be less apparent, so let's look at this aspect more closely.

Awareness and Acknowledgment

Becoming aware is the first move in taking a purposeful breathing space. The aim of this step is to use the power of mindfulness

- To disentangle ourselves from the doing, ruminative mode
- To drop into a feeling/sensing/knowing/being mode
- To acknowledge or witness our thoughts, feelings, and body sensations as we rest in awareness of them

Perhaps because the practice is called the "breathing space," the tendency is to go straight to the breath. But the first instruction does not even mention the breath. Instead, we are invited to become aware of our posture and intentionally allow it to express a sense of dignity, of taking a stand in our life, in our own body, to whatever degree may be possible in this moment. In this way we are "tuning the instrument" to prepare to step out of automatic pilot mode and to acknowledge whatever is going on right now. This stepping out of autopilot and into awareness is inextricably linked.

After we've prepared in this way, the instructions for Step 1 invite us to focus our attention inward and to acknowledge our experience of thoughts, feelings, and body sensations, *in turn*, in that very moment. We start with thoughts because, most often, that is where our minds are likely to be focused as we begin the breathing space. We focus on body sensations last, as this then provides a natural transition to focusing on the body sensations of breathing in Step 2. It may come as a surprise to know that this very act of parsing or sorting of experience into these three aspects—thoughts, feelings, and body sensations—is, in and of itself, of great importance. Although we may initially perceive an unpleasant experience as an undifferentiated "bad thing," a big black blob that we just want to be rid of, if we attend to it more closely, we will generally find that it can be recognized as an interlinked pattern of thoughts, feelings, and body sensations. Becoming aware of the separate components of the pattern in this way can be invaluable in and of itself—the mind will respond differently, in new and potentially more creative ways, to the perception of a complex mosaic of distinct experiences than it will to the perception of a uniform hated thing.

> Intentionally separating an unpleasant experience into thoughts, feelings, and body sensations allows the mind to respond more creatively than it would to the perception of an event as monolithic, impenetrable, and overwhelming.

Like many other participants in the program, Matthew first became aware of the power of parsing his experience while using the Pleasant and Unpleasant Events Calendar described in Chapter 6. Because he also happened to be a psychologist, Matthew knew very well intellectually that emotional experiences can be broken down into these three aspects. But as he undertook the simple exercise of attending to each component, he was staggered by the difference that it made to know this *experientially*. Suddenly he was able to *relate* to unpleasant experiences as simply bundles of thoughts, feelings, and body sensations. Identifying less personally with his response to unpleasant events, he found the whole situation became lighter, more spacious, freer. The first step of the three-minute breathing space provides a way to bring the same shift in perspective, to one degree or another, to any aspect of our experience.

The first step of the breathing space also provides an opportunity to *fully* acknowledge our experience in the moment, as Matthew discovered: "I was on a work trip, and my partner had come with me. The evening before the meeting, I was ironing some clothes, and my partner was reading on the other side of the room, behind me. I was tired and feeling a little anxious about how the next day would go. Was I sufficiently prepared?

"I found some resentment creeping into my mind. Here I was, ironing, when I could be preparing more for tomorrow, if she would only help me out a bit. There she was, just reading. I recognized this as a not-very-helpful thought stream—I think of myself as a 'modern man' who takes care of his own needs. I told myself that she had every right to be enjoying her holiday, and so it was appropriate for me to take responsibility for my own clothes. But somehow, a part of me did not seem satisfied with this. Soon another thought appeared. *But this is a very important meeting—and this is one occasion when I should not have to be ironing when I could be preparing. Why can't she see my predicament and offer to help me?* The resentment and irritation were rapidly mounting.

"The Vietnamese meditation teacher Thich Nhat Hanh talks about doing activities just to do them—for example, doing the dishes just to do the dishes (and not just to get them finished to rush on to the next activity). Here was a perfect opportunity to practice his teaching. Right. Focus on the ironing . . . the texture of the cloth, the smell of hot steam, the movement of the iron. Then the next thought arose: *No! I should not have to be using my mindfulness practice to cope with this ironing. I should not have to be doing the ironing at all.* I tried to focus again, gritting my mental teeth. *Focus on ironing, the smell of the steam, the feel of the cloth!* No use. The thoughts came streaming back.

"It was at that moment that I remembered the breathing space. The first step was not focusing but acknowledging. I became aware that I was trying to use meditation to change things; I had not acknowledged the situation in its entirety! Here was the ironing, here was the resentment, here were the thoughts. Acknowledging meant allowing all of it to be present as it was and, as the breathing space unfolded, to be able to say inwardly to myself: *It's okay for me to feel this: whatever it is, it's already here.* For me, this meant giving up the struggle to be 'good,' and to acknowledge that, at that moment, I felt really resentful—and to say *It's okay not to like feeling this way.* Of course this felt dangerous, as if it would allow my resentment to get out of hand.

"In fact, amazingly, it dropped away. Why? Because for the first time in that little scene, I guess I had acknowledged the whole thing: I had seen what was really happening, rather than obsessing about what I thought *should* be happening.

"As it turned out, I need not have been too concerned about preparing for the meeting. During that night, some people came into our hotel room as we slept and stole most of our possessions, including our computers, diaries, credit cards, and money. At the meeting the following day, somehow ironing, or how prepared I was, did not seem that important."

Matthew reported later that he had originally thought he was acknowledging what was going on and taking action. But then, he said, he realized that his acknowledgment was only partial. He recognized that he was attempting to use the practice to escape or fix or dispel his bad mood. The change in his mood came about only when he was first able and willing to hold *all* aspects of what was going on in awareness, including his resentment, with full acknowledgment. As we saw in Chapter 7, the shift from rejecting a situation or condition to accepting it as it is, *because* it is already as it is, is essential to responding skillfully to a difficult or unpleasant situation. Often, wholehearted acknowledgment of what is already present may actually be all that is necessary, as Matthew discovered for himself by staying with the process. The first step of the breathing space provides a structured, systematic way to do just that, namely, acknowledge wholeheartedly what is already the case. The second and third steps allow that shift in perspective to be consolidated and stabilized.

> Sometimes just acknowledging what's actually going on instead of dwelling on what "should" be happening is all that is needed to transform our experience.

Using the Breathing Space

We need to be cautious of a potential pitfall in the way we use the breathing space. It is easy to see it as merely a time-out, a brief moment when we can retreat and relax before advancing again into the busyness of our lives. Although it may have some short-term benefits along these lines, the time-out approach is not as helpful in the long run as the shift from doing to being mode because it does not alter our feelings of being under stress and pressure. It is best to see the breathing space as an opportunity to bring awareness to whatever is going on at this moment, to notice and step out of the routine we have become caught up in, so that we might relate differently to whatever difficulty we could be facing.

What is the difference between taking a break and taking a breathing space? An analogy may help. Most of us have at some time been caught in a severe downpour and have had to run for shelter. Sometimes we are simply glad to be out of the rain. We stand for a while, hoping it will stop. We are dry at the moment, but as the rain continues we know that sooner or later we are going to have to face it; the thing we tried to escape is still here. Finally, in one scenario, we go back out into the rain, grumbling, even cursing our luck as the rain drenches us.

At other times, another scenario might unfold for us. We may take shelter in a very different way. We stand in the dry for a while, aware of the prospect of getting soaked and not liking it much. We notice that we are hoping that it will stop but, seeing that it shows no sign of stopping, realize that being upset about it and worrying about how soaked we are going to get is only adding to our discomfort. So we stop clinging to the hope that it will stop raining and we enter the downpour, letting ourselves be drenched and accepting that this is what is happening at the moment. Approaching the situation in this way may allow us to experience the rain itself. We may notice that there is something rather compelling about the way it is splashing off everything it hits. The rain has not stopped. We may be getting wetter and wetter. But our relationship to what is happening has changed the whole experience.

The analogy of seeking shelter from a rainstorm evokes the markedly different ways in which any meditative practice can be used: either as a

> **Taking a breathing space is not just taking a break.**

clever way of hiding from difficult experiences, hoping that they will go away, or as a way of turning to face them, changing the way we relate to them. The breathing space is more than a time-out, a time when we take shelter, gritting our teeth and hoping the storm will pass. By stepping out of automatic pilot, we allow ourselves to hold, as objects of our attention, everything in the here and now. This includes our breath and body sensations and the jumble of our feelings and thoughts. As we do this, we may find that our awareness of these feelings or thoughts brings with it a fresh and transformative perspective. Suddenly, we are inhabiting a wider view of our experience rather than being so caught up in it. This was Elisa's experience of the breathing space. She found she could use it when she felt overwhelmed by things at work. The stepping out of autopilot, acknowledging what thoughts, feelings, and body sensations were around, was really helpful preparation before gathering attention to focus on the breath.

"I use it especially when there is pressure and things happening and I want to get centered. . . . Ah, there it is, my breath . . . and then I step into it. A couple of times in the last week I've had to do it intentionally after going into a mood almost involuntarily—a negative reaction, which is where my depression comes from usually, turning everything so black, so bad. And so to refocus myself out of this, I just stop for a second. I use it just to keep me right where I am—instead of reacting to the situation, to actually stay in it."

Elisa discovered that she does not have to react to her bad moods by assuming they are telling the truth about what is going to happen:

"In the past when I've felt overwhelmed, thinking I'll never get better; this is going to go on forever, I've thought, That's how it is going to be . . . it is all over now. Now it's different somehow . . . it means I can actually realize, Well, hang on; it's not over yet. In some cases it hasn't even started, so Let's just stick around and see what's actually going on—doing this instead of letting my head determine that for me."

It takes some practice for the three-minute breathing space to serve as an effective, practical way to pause and gather ourselves in the midst of troubling situations. That is why it is useful to begin by scheduling time for a breathing space at three specific times during the day, for a week. That can get us launched into using it not only at preprogrammed times but also whenever we feel we most need it, such as when we feel under particular stress.

The aim is for the three-minute breathing space to become an important vehicle for bringing the growing power of our formal meditation practice into our daily life. Although we call it the three-minute breathing space, it is important to see that the precise form and duration of the breathing space can be tailored to the constraints of any situation in which we find ourselves. We can experiment with different forms of breathing space as life demands, accommodating to the realities of where we are. If we can take ourselves to a quiet place, we can indulge in the luxury of a full three-minute mini-meditation, with eyes closed if we find that helpful. But if we are in the middle of an argument, stuck in a traffic jam, trapped in a difficult meeting, or find ourselves clicking from one site to another on the internet, we will need to accommodate, flexibly and creatively, to the realities we encounter. We might have to keep our eyes open, compress the sequence into less than one minute, or gather our scattered attention on our footfalls as we walk, rather than keep our focus on the breath. The most important thing is that we have some understanding of what we are intending to do; then we can experiment with as many ways of doing the breathing space as our life demands. Just keeping in mind that a breathing space is always available to us profoundly affects many aspects of our lives.

If the breathing space is practiced regularly, we may find that stepping out of automatic pilot, followed by intentionally implementing the three steps, becomes a great ally in bringing mindfulness into everyday life. It can help us deal skillfully with the difficult and distressing affairs of life and also to become more appreciative of the many positive features of our lives in all those moments that would otherwise pass us by.

NOT TRYING TO FIX THINGS

Like all meditation practices, the three-minute breathing space requires a kind of effort. But if we are too goal-oriented about it, our very striving may only increase our difficulties, as Tara discovered. In her case, it was because she perceived the breathing space as too short. "I was conscious that it should just be three minutes," she explained, "so it just feels like I have got to rush in there and think about—you know—what I've got to think about, settling down, and then I am sort of panicking that I am going to miss the three minutes. I can't relax. When I'm taking a coffee break and checking my phone—getting dragged down a rabbit hole reacting to somebody's reaction to a reaction—I realize what I'm doing, and I decide to take an emergency breathing space, but I'm too frazzled to connect with it."

The breathing space itself can actually become a source of aversion if it is practiced in the spirit of fixing things. Tara realized this on her own when she noticed that she was harboring an expectation that she had to "do it *right*" if it was to "work" to calm her down. She decided to take a different approach, saying to herself, *Okay, remember, there is no goal here. All I have to do is note inwardly what is going on—thoughts, feelings, body sensations—bring my mind to the breath and the belly, and then to a wider awareness including the body as a whole. If I do that, that's fine. I've done what I have to do. The rest will take care of itself.*

For Tara, as for any of us, our challenge and our responsibility in this practice is simply to give ourselves over to it as best we can, remembering that what matters is our orientation toward the present moment—*what we bring to it.* What we get out of it is not under our control. It is part of the adventure to observe compassionately, as best we can, and see what comes of stopping and dropping in on ourselves in this way in the midst of our daily lives. That is all. In this way, when we are plagued with thoughts such as *This is not working* or *I don't have the time* or *I'm obviously not doing it right,* we begin to see that *these thoughts are exactly what we need to become aware of and exactly what we need to acknowledge.* If we are motivated to undertake the challenge of waking up to our lives, we only need to remember to take the time to use the breathing space and then to give ourselves over to it, as best we can in any given moment. One way of expressing this is to say that each of us is responsible for the *input.* We do not need to worry about the *outcome,* especially about whether it is "working." The invitation is to be patient and to persevere in the practice and see what happens.

> As with all meditation practices, if we find ourselves setting goals for the breathing space, we'll revert from being mode back into doing mode.

As she practiced the breathing space for the next week, Tara decided that it was worth trying to bring to it a sense of *allowing.* She decided that she didn't have to "do it well" or achieve any particular result. Just putting it into practice would be enough. When she returned for the next session of the class, she was intrigued by what had happened. "I noticed sensations," she said. "Whether they were there all along and I didn't notice them or whether they are new, I don't know. But I can certainly feel the physical sensations of anxiety like I haven't felt before. My suspicion is that they were there all along."

At this stage in her account, it was not clear how things would turn out for Tara, but her experience did suggest that allowing the physical sensations of anxiety to be held in awareness gave her opportunities to know them in new ways, and thereby to see new aspects of them. She calls it their "ebb and flow."

"I think my body makes me aware of them," Tara said. "And then I can focus on them and, you know, feel what's going on. I had never really paid attention to what is going on physically before. I've certainly been familiar with paying attention to the thoughts, but never the sensations. That changes everything. It doesn't necessarily make things worse or better, but there is an ebb and flow, an ongoing change in texture and feeling."

The breathing space reminded Tara of one of the central messages of the whole mindfulness program: to learn how to relate differently to the constantly changing patterns in the mind and the body; to hold the recurrent patterns of both mind and body in the accepting and openhearted embrace of awareness, especially at those times when we feel tired or down or anxious, when the mind's reactivity and old habits are likely to be most overwhelming. Tara's words sum it up well: "I can see the value in noticing that it does ebb and flow and change on its own and that I don't have to fix it. It's being with it and not being more afraid of it."

WHEN THINGS ARE HECTIC

Hana's experience was very similar to Tara's. She found she could practice the breathing space when she was calm, but she found it much more difficult when things got hectic. Hana works in a large department store: "It's easy when I'm relatively calm. It is also okay when you can see a bad big black cloud coming and take yourself in hand and do it. But yesterday and today, I have been really busy. Everybody's been rushed, and I've been going backward and forward and up and down the escalator."

When everything is hectic like this for Hana, the meditation practice becomes drawn, unwittingly, into the whirlpool along with everything else she has to do, and she criticizes herself for not remembering to use it. "It's been awful," she said, "and I should have been breathing and steadying myself, but it was all too frantic, and I didn't even think about it today. Things overtook me."

In making "shoulds" for herself, Hana's doing mind is importing tension into any decision she might make about whether to practice or not. Instead of simply practicing a three-minute breathing space when the impulse arises, she ends up only *thinking* about it. Here we see the doing mode in all its splendor: measuring the gap between how things are and how they "should be" and then trying to close the gap. The practice has become a victim of thinking and striving.

MINDFULNESS IS INVITING AND FORGIVING

We now arrive at the critical point. It seems easiest to be mindful at the times when we least need it. Then, when we most need it, our capacity to meet the moment with mindfulness seems to evaporate. If we wish to sidestep this vicious cycle, we need to build up new attitudes to counterbalance our old habits. Whenever we feel hassled, *that* is the perfect moment to take a breathing space. Even if we only manage to do it after the fact, rather than during whatever is happening, this will help us build new ways of seeing, knowing, and responding to stressful situations. This might mean taking a breathing space *after* that aggravating phone call if not during it or while we're rehashing some difficult incident that we wish had gone differently. So even if we realize at the end of the day *Oh my gosh—it's eight o'clock at night, and I haven't actually been in touch with my body or the breath once today*, there and then, right in that moment, as soon as we become aware of it, we can take a breathing space. *That moment is a moment of realization and is now the perfect moment to practice and to implement the breathing space.* Without our having to worry about it or force it, the practice itself will influence, in ways both little and not-so-little, our relationship to how our life is unfolding. With continued practice, the habits of a lifetime of operating in the doing mode will attenuate and dissolve in the spacious, accepting embrace of mindfulness. In this way, each time we take a breathing space we are building up increments of a new learning. So even if we think *Oh, I haven't done my practice for several days,* we can seize that very moment and practice. We may think *There's no point; I've missed too much; I might as well pack it in, give up.* Those thoughts can then serve as our cue, as a reminder to practice. Otherwise, a spiral of rumination has an opportunity to take hold right then and there as we berate ourselves for not doing what we are "supposed" to be doing. Ironically, that cycle of rumination might last at least three minutes!

One more instance of being subverted by the "coulda, shoulda, woulda, oughta" mentality—or choosing not to be.

> Whenever we feel hassled, it is helpful to take a breathing space— even if after the fact.

Mindfulness practice is very forgiving. It beckons to us to start over again, time after time after time, without judging us for the times we haven't managed to remember to drop in on ourselves. So we do it whenever and wherever we can, as a gesture of kindness toward ourselves. This orientation and an ongoing willingness to practice now, whatever happened or didn't happen in that regard in the past, will strengthen the likelihood that the next time we really "need" to be fully present, the breathing space will immediately suggest itself as a skillful option.

Choices We Can Make after Taking a Breathing Space

It is helpful to think of the breathing space as a door through which we can pass from the hot, murky, cramped, "driven" places in our minds to a lighter, cooler, more accommodating space. If we see the breathing space as always the first step in a more mindful response to unpleasant feelings of unhappiness, anger, fear, and the like, then our initial focus need only be on that one door. But once through that door, once we have entered a different space in our minds, a number of other doors lie before us, leading onward. Each door offers a different option for further mindful responding, and we are invited to make a conscious choice of which door to open next. Our choices may be severely constrained by the situation in which we find ourselves. Even so, we always have the option of returning later to these possibilities to expand and deepen our practice.

OPTION 1: REENTRY

The simplest option after we've completed the third step of the breathing space is to leave it at that. With a new mode of mind in place, we mentally reenter the difficult situation that prompted us to take the breathing space. We may find the negative thoughts, the unpleasant feelings, the intense physical sensations, the shouting boss, or the screaming child are all still here. But the fact that we can approach them now in being mode, from a gathered, deliberate, more spacious, and less self-centered perspective can make all the difference.

We can now approach them matter-of-factly, responding skillfully to the needs of the moment, rather than automatically reacting in ways that will simply compound the difficulties we experience. Once we are in this mode of mind, its inherent wisdom may make the next step we need to take much clearer. And we can support this wiser mode by staying mindfully present, as best we can, *grounded in awareness of our bodily experience in each moment.*

Sometimes the change is very subtle. One participant reported: "On Wednesday I woke up feeling rotten. I hadn't slept well; I was tired and thick-headed. I had a day of work ahead of me. I could feel the old familiar feelings of desperation rising up. As I was lying there feeling miserable, some part of me remembered my breath, and I took a breathing space. After it, I lay in bed for a while just watching my breath and tuning in to the sensations in my body. It seems odd, but I felt different after that—I still felt tired, thick-headed, and fed up, but it didn't seem like such a disaster!"

Although the shift in feeling tone may be a subtle one, it actually represents a huge and crucial change in mode of mind. And every tiny shift of this kind, no matter how subtle, can open up new possibilities for what happens next.

It may mean working on our to-do list one task at a time, rather than getting overwhelmed by all the things left undone. It may mean ending a frustrating phone call feeling aggravated but not demeaned or disrespected. It could mean feeling regretful about snapping at a colleague without having the feeling that we should beat ourselves up over it again and again during the rest of the day. Maybe it means just feeling down when something reminds us of a recent loss or disappointment but not adding anger at the situation or ourselves, nor descending into feeling "I'll never get over this," which can so quickly empty the present and the future of all hope.

Of course, we always have the option, if time permits, of building on this new learning by going around again: taking another breathing space to consolidate the shift to the new, more mindful, mode of mind. But the danger here is that we could end up approaching the breathing space in a goal-oriented way—as a tool to "fix" a difficult situation. From this perspective, if the first breathing space did not "work" in getting rid of unwanted feelings, we might be tempted to try again, perhaps even harder this time. The risk here is that the attempt to fix things actually becomes a part of the problem. The "failure" of the first and possibly subsequent attempts to get rid of negative feelings generates more negative feelings. This is the exact opposite of mindfulness.

> If we choose to repeat the breathing space, we have to make sure we're not trying to use it as a quick fix—the opposite of mindfulness.

We may find that we need to explicitly remind ourselves quite frequently that the aim of the three-minute breathing space is not to dispose of all negative states, instantly or otherwise, but to allow us to access a mode of mind in which we can be with them more effectively and with greater clarity. Although this may not immediately eliminate whatever it is that we don't want to continue happening, it will give us the freedom and wisdom to respond in ways that may allow unpleasant feelings and difficult situations to resolve rather than perpetuate themselves. At the very least, we can cease feeding them and compounding the suffering.

If we wish to explore the option of using several breathing spaces back to back, it might be wise to limit ourselves to two cycles of it on any one occasion. *We might keep in mind that the breathing space, used properly, is merely a method for reminding us of what it would mean and how it would feel to embody mindfulness in the face of whatever is arising.*

OPTION 2: THE BODY DOOR

As we have emphasized many times, disturbing experiences carry an unpleasant feeling tone. There are negative feelings, such as dread or sadness, and often a reaction of aversion or resistance to them, not uncommonly expressed in changes in the muscles of the face or body, such as frowning; tightening of the neck, jaw, and shoulder muscles; or tensing of the lower back. All of these can be directly attended to, and our primary strategy for transforming our relationship to difficult emotions is to work within this domain of awareness (Chapter 7). So if, following an initial breathing space, we choose to work further on our emotions, it is natural to turn our attention toward what we are feeling in the body.

As a first step we direct, as best we can, a friendly, open attention to the part of the body where we experience the most intense physical bodily sensations. One way to do this is to use the breath to carry the attention, breathing into the area on each in-breath, breathing out from the area on each out-breath, as we learned to do in the body scan. With each out-breath, any sense of tightness, bracing, or resistance may release or soften naturally. Where this occurs, the tension and sense of holding on often dissolve with the out-breath, although by no means are we trying to *make* this happen. If it happens, that's fine, but it's equally fine if it does not. The simple act of bringing awareness to the sense of aversion and resistance is enough, without becoming fixated on achieving relaxation. We may find it helpful to remind ourselves of the general intention to allow and accept our experience by saying in our minds *Softening, opening, embracing.*

> The tension we notice in a particular area of the body may naturally soften with the out-breath, if we don't try to force it to do so.

Once we have brought attention to the physical, bodily manifestations of any resistance or aversion we may be feeling, we can explore a number of options for staying connected with our feelings. Staying in touch with them allows for the possibility of their being met and held in new and different ways. One is simply to continue breathing with awareness of the sensations, perhaps having the sense of holding them in a soft, wide, and spacious awareness. Another option is to investigate in detail, with a narrower, intentionally more focused attention, where the area of intensity begins; where its edges are; where the sensations are most intense; how, if at all, the sensations change from one moment to the next. Whatever option we choose, we expend some effort to keep our awareness alive and to nurture it. We can do this by intentionally infusing it with qualities of interest, investigation, goodwill, and compassion. If we find that we have drifted into an attitude of forcing or striving, we can gently but firmly disengage from it. Plus, we can always refresh and enliven our minds by opening and widening the field of awareness to include other senses in the moment such as sounds, the fragrance of the air, or the feeling of the air on the skin.

We can approach any negative feelings in the same way. We may find it helpful to remind ourselves to cultivate an accepting, allowing relationship to these feelings by saying to ourselves *It's okay for me to feel this; whatever it is, it's already here.* We might pay particular attention to any changes in the qualities of those feelings as we hold them in awareness.

With intensely unpleasant feelings, we may find it helpful to use the strategy of "working the edge." As explained earlier, this means bringing attention as far into the intensity of the experience as we can and then maintaining it with a light touch, as best we can, moment by moment. When the intensity begins to feel overwhelming, we can gently, in the spirit of self-compassion, shift our attention bit by bit toward some other, more stabilizing and benign focus. For instance, we might steady ourselves and regroup by focusing on the movements of the breath until we feel ready to approach the area of greater intensity again. We can do this by focusing on the breath by itself or together with awareness of the unpleasant feelings and sensations in the background ("breathing with"). By testing the water in this way, we can develop a progressively more accepting relationship to intensely unpleasant experiences. This in itself is a path of both wisdom and compassion.

Michelle found herself feeling drained just thinking about an upcoming family reunion. "I keep telling myself that it should be nice to visit with everyone after all this time," she said, "but when I think of making the travel arrangements, I can't seem to follow through." Back at home the next day, the thought *I should get it all booked* came into her mind once again. Instead of forcing herself to search online right then and there, she decided she would first take a breathing space. A few minutes into it, Michelle noticed increased pressure in her chest and tightness in her throat. The thought that her father would be coming to the reunion with his new partner seemed to increase the intensity of these sensations. Ordinarily, Michelle would have turned away from looking at this thought pattern more closely, telling herself that it was up to her to "do the right thing for the family." This time, however, she was able to recognize her aversion as being an all too familiar response and decided, instead, to approach the edge of her discomfort. Once she had connected with her breath at the belly, she moved her attention to her throat and began to breathe into the tightness. What she discovered was that these sensations were not static: they came and went. The tightness gave way to a feeling of strain in her neck muscles, and this would sometimes ease as she breathed out from this region. She noticed that the thought *You ought to welcome her into the family* was quickly followed by *How could he be so insensitive? It's only been six months since Mom passed away.* Now her throat felt slightly blocked and squeezed. Still, she continued breathing as anger and hurt registered in her mind, and then sadness and loss over her mother. "Even though I don't know what I'll end up doing," she said, "just letting this stuff in right now is a way that I can care for myself. Maybe that's a start." Given what we now know about how rumination actively inhibits sensory processing, the small opening to body sensations that Michelle experienced might have been the start of an important healing process.

> Working the edge is a good way to test the water when an experience is so unpleasant that aversion is likely to take over.

OPTION 3: THE THOUGHT DOOR

In the first step of the breathing space we may become aware that emotionally charged thoughts are the most salient feature of our experience. From Chapter 8, we may recognize among these some of our recurring patterns of negative thoughts. If these thoughts are still a dominant feature of our experience as we complete Step 3 of the breathing space, we have the option of opening the thought door by making a deliberate decision to relate differently to our thinking. This may involve

- Writing down the thoughts
- Watching the thoughts come and go
- Viewing the thoughts as mental events rather than as facts
- Relating to thoughts in the same way that we would to sounds
- Identifying a particular thought pattern as one of our recurring old mental grooves

▪ Gently asking ourselves:
   Am I overtired?
   Am I jumping to conclusions?
   Am I thinking in black-and-white terms?
   Am I expecting perfection?

The key idea is that, based on our previous experience of meditation practice, we probably will have already discovered some effective ways to relate differently and more creatively to negative thoughts when they arise. In the breathing space, we can now make use of those various approaches to remind ourselves that we are not our thoughts and that thoughts are not facts (even the ones that say they are!). This reminder alone can have profound effects that accumulate over time.

This is what Malik discovered. As a teenager living in a large city, he'd really enjoyed the social life, celebrating with friends and family and going out a lot. And then 9/11 happened. Things changed. His commute on the subway in the months and years afterward was totally different from what it had been before. He found he couldn't run for a sliding door for fear people might think the worst. Every commute, he sensed his body tense, contracted and wound up. He became depressed.

This particular day the car was crowded and someone had barged into him by accident and he'd fallen sideways. As he got up again, he felt as if all eyes were on him and on the bag he was carrying. By the time he got home he was exhausted. Another evening of no energy, of staying in, of ordering food and eating alone.

Malik knew there was a seed of reality to his feelings, at least all those years ago—but now? He was well aware of the tension, sadness, and exhaustion he had been carrying over these many years. Now the MBCT practice was gradually helping him explore his thoughts. He began to see that what was making his feelings persist always started with the thought that everyone was looking at him: "It's obvious everyone thinks I'm dangerous. Things will never be the same again. It's ruined my whole life."

His formal practice at home had begun to help him see thoughts, feelings, and sensations from a wider perspective, and now he decided to use the breathing space as a portable practice to use right when he needed it—on the subway. He would do the whole three steps, taking time over the first step to acknowledge the "weather pattern" in mind and body at that moment without trying to change it. This, he found, already gave him the glimmer of hope that the situation might be workable. After a while, when he felt ready, he would gather his attention and focus on his breath, sometimes including the sensations of his feet on the floor as well, then widening his attention to the body as a whole. With the body in the background, he opened the thought door: "Okay—let's watch the thoughts come and go. Here they are—I recognize these: *People think I'm bad. I can't stand this. Nothing will be the same.* I began to view my thoughts in the same way that I was hearing the sounds of the subway. Because there were so many sounds, I could easily switch my focus between sounds and thoughts; this really helped me see my thoughts as events coming and going in my mind, rather than as the absolute truth. I could see the vicious circle I was trapped in—my tension was feeding the thoughts, and they were feeding the tension. And yes, I could see that being tired at the end of the day was not helping; it was making everything seem more catastrophic and permanent.

"At first things began to change, but by very little. Then one day I opened my eyes and saw a child across the car smiling at me. And I found myself smiling back—and her dad smiled too. I got talking to him, and he said they were visiting from South Africa. And I looked round, and I saw so many people—different ages, colors, hairstyles, clothes, different everything! And I thought *Here is another rainbow nation in this subway, right now.*"

OPTION 4: THE DOOR OF SKILLFUL ACTION

A fourth choice we can make after the breathing space is to open the door of skillful action. We have emphasized the importance of bringing an accepting and allowing awareness to difficult and unpleasant experiences (Chapter 7). But this new orientation does *not* mean we have to be passive. Often, the most appropriate response to unpleasant feelings, once we have acknowledged them, will be to take some considered action, to act on the basis of conscious choice.

The motivation underlying our actions at these times will determine whether they turn out to be helpful or unhelpful. As we saw in the mouse-in-the-maze experiment (Chapter 6), the same action can have very different consequences depending on whether our motivation is based on avoidance or on openness to experience. If we are driven to get rid of the unpleasant feelings, our actions will most likely backfire, digging us deeper into unhappiness. On the other hand, if we are motivated by genuine desire to take better care of ourselves, our actions can be a skillful way to bring greater ease and relief.

Betty used the breathing space to find some more room for her needs in a pressure-filled job. As an accountant, she felt herself most vulnerable around tax season and at the end of the fiscal year. This often meant long days and weekends at the office with little downtime. Recognizing that her last depression started under these circumstances, Betty made a point of going out in the afternoon to get a cup of her favorite coffee concoction and would drink it while sitting on one of those tall barstools watching the other customers. Sometimes she would pick up dinner at her neighborhood taqueria to get some relief from cooking at home. "In the past, I'd postpone going out until the pile of work I had to face was done," she said. "What's new is that I realize, 'now and not later': that I need to slow down and take time for myself in the moments that really matter."

Low mood particularly affects two sorts of activity: It makes the things we used to find pleasurable less enjoyable, causing us to lose interest in them or to give them up altogether. It also makes it difficult to stay on top of the daily tasks of living that may not give us pleasure but do give us a sense of being responsible people exercising control in our own lives. In many ways, subtle and not so subtle, depression and low mood undermine us by robbing us of the energy to do the things that would nourish us the most. Simply engaging or reengaging in such activity can have unsuspected power.

So the fourth possibility following a breathing space is to intentionally choose to do something that would once have given us (a) pleasure (such as having a hot bath, going for a walk with the dog, visiting a friend, listening to music that makes us feel good) or (b) a sense (no matter how small) of mastery, satisfaction, achievement, or control (such as clearing out a cupboard or drawer; doing something that we have been putting off, such as paying a bill, writing a letter to a family member or a friend, clearing off a desktop). Even a tiny amount of one such activity can give us a sense that we can have an effect in the world. And even a small effect can counteract the sense of helplessness and lack of control that often accompanies low mood. In the case of very anxious, fearful moods, it may be particularly helpful to take action by facing and taking on situations that we have hitherto avoided. It's also both skillful and realistic to break tasks down into smaller steps and tackle only one step at a time. In all cases, it's very helpful to remember to congratulate ourselves for completing a task or even the smallest part of a task.

In exploring the most effective way to take action in responding mindfully to a depressed mood, it may be helpful to keep two things in mind. First, *low mood undermines and reverses the motivation process itself.* Normally we can wait until we want to do something, and then just do it. However, when we feel low, we actually have to mobilize ourselves to do something *before* we want to do it. Second, the tiredness and fatigue that occur in depression can be misleading. When we are not depressed, tiredness means we need to rest. In this case, rest refreshes us. *The fatigue of depression, however, is often not normal tiredness; it may call not for rest but for increased activity, if only for a short while.* Rest can worsen the fatigue. The invitation here is to see for ourselves what's true for us. What do we notice when we take a rest? What do we notice when we respond by increasing activity? Part of taking care of ourselves when depression threatens to switch off all our motivation is to stay in the flow of life, to keep participating in normal activities, even if our mood and thoughts seem to say there's no point.

The most challenging times are often when depression comes out of the blue, such as on waking up. Here too our initial response can be to start by taking a breathing space. It is also important to ask some specific questions:

- "How can I best be kind to myself right now?"
- "What is the best gift I can give to myself at this moment?"
- "I do not know how long this mood will last so how can I best look after myself until it passes?"
- "What would I do at this moment for someone I cared about who was feeling this way? How can I look after myself in the same way?"

Of course, even with the best of intentions, sometimes we won't be able to catch ourselves; it may feel that we have gone over an edge, into a more persistent and intense negative mood state. At such times it's important that, however weakly or fleetingly, we remember that the practice of mindfulness is still a healthy way to take care of ourselves. Recent research shows that MBCT can help here too; that what we need at such times is actually no different from what we find helpful in responding mindfully to our less intense negative moods. Of course, it may be more challenging to relate differently to our negative thoughts in such moments. Perhaps even the impact of engaging in some mood-lifting activity may be severely muted under the circumstances. Nevertheless *it is still better to bring whatever degree of mindfulness we can to this moment and take some appropriate action to care for ourselves than to sink further into a state of ruminative brooding.*

What we are saying here is that the task, when things are tough, is really to focus on each moment: to handle each moment as best we can. If our approach to how we relate to a difficult moment shifts even by 1 percent, that is potentially an enormous shift to have made because it affects the next moment, and the next moment, and so on; so one seemingly small change can have a surprisingly large impact down the road.

The Freedom to Choose

In reflecting on what he had learned from his participation in the mindfulness program, Louis singled out the way in which he found the breathing space to be an important ally:

"I realized many things, but one I'd like to share. I've realized how much I really push myself. This is something I know how to do really well. So I spent lots of time thinking about how I would be able to recognize it. The three-minute breathing space helps a lot. And I am doing it a number of times throughout the day. Sometimes three times, sometimes five times, sometimes whenever there is a big hesitation or not knowing . . . or when there are still six more things left to do and I have half an hour or an hour left to go; that's when it's really great. It really helps me . . . just to sit . . . to do this acknowledgment . . . and then to hold this 'not knowing' . . . because sometimes I really don't know where this feeling of pressure comes from. Do I really have to push myself and say that in the next half an hour I will finish the project? Sometimes I just stay with *I don't know* . . . and it's okay not to know, and it's okay also for me not to take an action to finish everything. Because it's so easy for me to take an action, and that's where a lot of stress in my life comes from, just from taking too many actions, having too many things on my plate and doing it all . . . because I feel I won't go to sleep unless I do this so everything is finished. I have to know it's completed. And sometimes it's just not necessary. This is very new for me . . . *not* to do certain things . . . and it feels okay. In a way I'm also changing my attitude toward time. The time that I have, the time I can give myself for doing something, you know? I think I am less frantic because of that."

Louis was raising a very important point. There's no simple way to answer the question of what different people need. Some of us who are too busy may need to find a balance that involves stepping away from endless activity. Others might find we're not doing enough of the things we need to be doing, and so the problem is finding a way of balancing our lives so that we can be more engaged and enlivened at certain times. One way to begin is to bring awareness to where we are and to the feeling of what is going on with us right now. This gives us more sensitivity to appraise our inner and outer situation and condition accurately—not just cerebrally, but through mindful awareness. This awareness in turn expands the field of choices available to us and increases the likelihood that we will make healthy, wise, skillful choices rather than be carried along by the momentum of what we habitually do.

The expansion of choices may be instantaneous and unexpected, as Kat found out when she picked up her fifteen-year-old son from school after having been away for a few days.

"I had forgotten how grumpy fifteen-year-olds can be," she said. "I asked him how school had been that day. He said angrily, 'You always say the same thing.'

"I paused, and I was aware of a feeling of contraction in my chest. It was very distinct. I recognized rising tension and irritation. I would normally have reacted."

For Kat, somehow, just that pause, that instantaneous acknowledgment, gathering, and awareness of the body, was enough to let the moment pass without reacting.

"I would usually have gotten angry at him or driven home in a cold silence," Kat went on. "Instead, I turned to him and found myself saying 'I've missed you.' And you know what? He turned to me and smiled. I had not seen that smile in ages. It was a miracle."

The three-minute breathing space is intended to provide us with just that kind of sensitivity and potential for choice when we come face to face with old patterns. These old patterns may relate to thinking about ourselves in a certain way or dealing with our moods in unhealthy ways or keeping ourselves insanely busy while blaming it on outside circumstances. Those habitual tendencies are still going to be here; mindfulness practice will not instantly change all that. But what it can do is to give us a moment's pause and present us with choices we had not seen before. Our starting point can be centered with the breath, fully acknowledging where we are now, right in this moment. Otherwise we can just be carried away as we always have been, reacting automatically. This is what Louis was realizing.

"I actually appreciate this state of not knowing," he explained. "I really do. Because it gives me a way of really pausing, and it opens my mind into right now. And somehow there is a moment when an idea comes to me and then I say yes or no. But also, holding it in awareness is somehow important, rather than just doing something automatically, which is what I would tend to do."

In practicing using the breathing space regularly, we gradually see that there is a way of changing our relationship to ourselves and the world. We find we can have a new relationship to aspects of ourselves that we previously found difficult and a new relationship to situations that we have been avoiding. Internal or external, these situations tend to evoke the same reaction in us: avoidance, escape, suppression. So as not to succumb to these unwise maneuvers, we *turn toward* whatever it is that has evoked these reactions. Because our habitual reactions of aversion to what we find difficult are fundamental to what gets us stuck in unhappiness, this conscious response of turning toward such difficulties, even if merely a one-degree turn in this direction, can bring about a fundamental shift in the way we live our lives.

Part IV

Reclaiming Your Life

Ten

Fully Alive

FREEING YOURSELF
FROM CHRONIC UNHAPPINESS

> People say that what we're all seeking is a meaning for life.
> I don't think that's what we're really seeking. I think that
> what we're seeking is an experience of being alive.
> —JOSEPH CAMPBELL, *The Power of Myth*

In *Frog and Toad Together,* a children's book that speaks as much to adults as to children, Arnold Lobel recounts a day in the life of Toad. Upon awakening, Toad sat up in bed and jotted a to-do list for the day on a piece of paper. It included activities like waking up, which he immediately crossed off since, well, he was already awake. Next on his schedule were routine activities like having breakfast and putting on his clothes. He then added heading out to Frog's home, where they could go for a walk together, followed by lunch, napping, playing games, eating again, and then retiring for the night. Before he did anything, he consulted his list and then announced that they would now engage in that activity. Every time he completed one of the items on his list he crossed it off. Then, at one point, disaster struck: a strong wind blew the list out of Toad's hand. Frog was all for running after the list to catch it. But poor Toad just could not do that—it was not on his list of things to do! So, while Toad sat there, immobilized, Frog ran after the list, mile after mile—but in vain—he just could not catch it and returned empty-handed to the disconsolate Toad. Toad could not remember any of the things that were left on his list to do. So he just sat and did nothing. Frog sat with him. Eventually Frog pointed out that it was getting dark and they should go to sleep. This idea triggered Toad's memory of the last item on his list. Bedtime! Delighted that he could, at last, cross out his whole day, Toad picked up a stick and scratched *going to sleep* into the ground. Then he crossed it out with great satisfaction, and he and Frog went to sleep.

Poor One-Mode Toad! Yet many of us often behave just like Toad, as if doing were the only mental mode available to us. Too often our lives seem to be little more than one long "to do" list.

It is not so much making "to do" lists that is the problem. The problem is our sense of impending doom if we don't get through the list. That, and the myopic narrowing of our lives that can result. Take Sam, for example, who was taking the MBCT program because of persistent and recurring low mood that was draining all the joy from his life. Early in the program he'd been skeptical, but a discussion in one of the classes about the driven-doing mode, and how hard it was to disengage from it, really struck home. He had started to look out for times when he found himself caught in one of the many "to do" lists that seemed to dominate his life.

Late one evening he found himself still at his desk, trying to finish a report for work he'd told himself he needed to finish that day. In fact, the deadline was not until the following week, but having set the goal, he was determined to meet it. He thought the final amendments to the document would be easy, but then it became clear that there was more to the task than he had imagined, compounded by the fact that his laptop had "updated" last week with a new and unfamiliar version of the software he used for his reports. His parents' advice from years ago came to mind—*leave it; you'll be fresher in the morning*—but as a point of principle he felt he must finish. With hunched shoulders and a frown on his face his fingers pecked at the keyboard long after his wife had said she was turning in for the night.

As he tried to save a chunk of new text, his work of the last half-hour disappeared from view. As his tension and frustration threatened to overwhelm him, he remembered the discussion in class, and paused, felt his feet on the floor, and allowed his attention to rest lightly on his breath as it moved into and out of his body. This calmed him down. But more than this. With a greater sense of calm, he saw something more clearly than he had before: that his *thoughts were just thoughts*—even those thoughts telling him he absolutely must complete this task because it was on his "to do" list. He realized how tense his shoulders were, and how tired his eyes, and found himself bringing a kindly awareness to them, then widening aware-ness to his whole body as he sat. And with this wider awareness of the being mode came a profound sense of intimacy toward himself, his body and mind, imbued with love and care. He saved his work, closed his laptop, and went to bed. He said later that this had been a turning point for him, and his enthusiasm for mindfulness practice had been firm from that point on.

Living his life ruled by his "to do" lists harmed Sam's health and well-being in countless ways. When those of us who struggle with relent-less unhappiness allow our interior worlds to be ruled by our "to do" lists, our emotional health is damaged. This puts our very lives at risk. Not only is driven-doing ineffective at staving off depression, but it constricts and cramps our lives so that we end up living in a tiny corner of the world avail-able to us.

Although we may not fully realize it, as human beings, every single one of us can live in the open spaciousness of the being mode far, far, more than we do. The more we make that possibility real for ourselves, even in tiny ways, the more we can enrich our own lives and enhance our mental health. Is it not wise, then, to reserve our use of the doing mode for those areas of life in which it is a skillful, effective response, and instead put more of our energies into the cultivation of being? This more mindful way of being takes some time and courage of course. But we can draw significant encourage-ment and inspiration from those who have engaged in exactly this kind of interior work through their participation in MBCT, keeping in mind that those formal programs lasted *only eight weeks* and reduced the risk of relapse by half in people who had been the most recurrently depressed.

"In situations in the past that would have knocked me sideways, or irri-tated me very much, I would have got upset about it and worked up— that just doesn't happen so often. It's been amazing the things that have happened in this short period—to stay calm without spiraling out of control."

"I've really learned to notice the early signs of my mood going down. For instance, when I put my phone down when I've been scrolling, then pick it up again a moment later without thinking, saying to myself 'Someone must have messaged me!' and then feel like trash—not only because I've been on my phone too long; I know that doesn't help, but also I feel, well, a bit lonely. Very soon I hear myself say *No one wants to know me.* I recognize that voice. I first heard it when I was fourteen, but now ten years later, I see it for what it is."

"Before I came here I didn't know what it was like to live without pressure. I might have had some idea when I was five years old, but I can't remember much of that. I have been shown a different way, and it's so simple. It seems to me *So that's what everybody else does all the time.* Nobody bothered to let me in on it before."

"It's the fact that I know the mindfulness skills are here, instead of having to rely on anybody else's helping hand and then feeling like a failure because I couldn't do it by myself. It's the fact that now I know there's something in me that gives me a handle on myself and the things that happen."

"I've been in this [prison] for six months now and still don't know when the appeal will come up. In here the noise is deafening and can go on all night. This course has helped me to be OK with loud noises and stress. It's helped my mind to stop racing, I can take a step back and take in the air around me. It's helped me in steadying myself when things are rushing in my head—concentrating on me now rather than what could be or has been. It helps me be more sensitive—for example [with] eating. Maybe it's like a guide to getting your senses back."

Our theories, our research, and the stories of other people's experience in their mindfulness programs all point to the importance of cultivating awareness intentionally. But in the end, all of this is still no substitute for *personal* experience. We each need to see for ourselves the effects of both the doing mode and the being mode on the moment-to-moment quality of our lives. To develop such experience requires that we cultivate mindfulness in our daily lives, for that is the arena in which most of our anguish arises and is played out. It is in the conduct and interactions of our everyday lives that we have a chance to become more aware of the consequences of the runaway doing mode and also to feel firsthand the transformative possibilities of dropping into being.

Ultimately, living with mindful awareness, grounded in the being mode of mind, is a way of being fully awake, fully alive, and fully oneself, whatever and however that might turn out to be. It doesn't prevent us from getting things done or bringing about important changes in our lives or in the world. It is very much about wise doing, a doing that emerges and flows out of the domain of being—"mindful doing" if you will. First we recognize our experience as being just as it is. Then, if we choose, we might intentionally engage in some appropriate action to take care of ourselves or respond compassionately to the particular situation, as the following three people did, each in their own way.

Peggy's Story

Peggy worked in a demanding job, advising caregivers in several different settings how best to handle their most difficult cases. Every morning she would wake with a feeling of dread and immediately begin worrying about how she was going to cope with the problems she had to confront that day. The specifics changed from day to day, but the underlying theme was always the same: fear that she would not be able to come up with answers to the difficulties presented to her, that things would get out of control, that she would not meet expectations, that everything would go dreadfully wrong and she would be to blame. On the worst days, the specific worries would trigger recurrent, more generalized feelings of fear. She would feel her heart sink at the bleak prospects before her: *Oh, God, it's always going to be like this. I'll never be able to hack it; it will always continue; I'll never feel free or relaxed.*

Before she encountered mindfulness training, Peggy had tried to deal with these worries by getting some sense of control over the specific problems that were uppermost in her mind each day as she lay in bed. She would identify the worry, anticipate what could go wrong, think what she could do to prevent it, reassure herself that she had done all that was necessary, or plan new ways to fix the problem and avoid the situations she feared and dreaded so much. Sometimes this approach seemed to take the edge off Peggy's fear. But there was no lasting effect. The next morning she would wake up in just as much dread, worried about a new set of problems.

What did Peggy do differently as a result of her mindfulness training?

212 ■ RECLAIMING YOUR LIFE

First, she concentrated on bringing attention to her body even before getting out of bed. She became aware of sensations of tension in the stomach and of an overall stiffness in the body, around the tension, as if she were already resisting it. Next she focused her attention on what she was feeling: the dread, the fear, the anxiety. With that came an awareness of just how unpleasant these feelings were, how much she hated them and wanted to be rid of them, and, with a sigh, a realization of just how drained and weary these feelings made her.

Through cultivating mindfulness, Peggy discovered that when she widened her attention to include the full scope of her experience in the moment, she was able to identify and distinguish four different aspects of her experience: (1) unpleasant physical sensations in the body; (2) unpleasant feelings, such as dread and fear; (3) previously unspoken negative thoughts about the feelings; and (4) the worries centered on the particular problems of the day.

Inspired by this wider perspective, Peggy made a crucial shift in the way she related to her difficulties. Rather than struggling with her feared images of the future, generated by all her worrying, Peggy reoriented herself to face the present reality and the actuality of her experiences in the moment. She realized that trying to solve the worries could never provide a long-term solution because, as one worry was put to rest, another would very quickly pop up to take its place.

> A little kindness and gentleness toward yourself is a wiser and more skillful response to feeling threatened than any amount of analytical problem solving.

Instead, Peggy settled into a practice she developed for herself. Each morning, she turned to face whatever experience awaited her as she woke up. She would greet the horrible lump in her stomach or throat, fully acknowledging how bad it felt: "There you are; I see you." Then, not running or turning away from it, she would explore the horrible feeling as a *feeling*. What was it like? What other feelings were here with it? She would acknowledge that the presence of the feeling meant there was something somewhere that she was perceiving as threatening. But, and here was a major shift, she no longer concerned herself with the particulars of the threat. She did not try fixing a difficult or threatening imagined situation in the future. Now, instead, her primary aim became to respond with greater awareness and acceptance to the immediate, present situation of *feeling threatened*. With this shift she recognized that kindness and gentleness, rather than analytical problem solving, were what was actually required—*You don't need to know what the details are this morning—the details don't matter. What matters is kindness and gentleness toward yourself.*

Peggy found that the dread still came, but it came less often, and when it did come she was able to be matter-of-fact with it. Rather than calling her experience of fear and dread "wrong" or interpreting it as a sign that she was deficient or that there was something profoundly wrong with her life, she now saw the feeling as a message reminding her of the need to be gentle, the need to be kind, the need to take good care of herself in a stressful time.

This is the shift in mode that we have been pointing to in this book. Like the novice in Chapter 4 (pages 72–74), Peggy had seen for herself that trying to make unpleasant thoughts and feelings go away by attempting to fix them or shut them out did not help her. It only increased her sense of helplessness. Her worries had constantly sucked her back in because she thought they ought to be solvable. Her mind kept activating the doing mode: fixing, analyzing, judging, comparing. Now she could identify the whole driven-doing mind pattern and see it as an opportunity to switch into being mode. She realized that with gentle persistence she could pay attention, intentionally, in each present moment of now to whatever she was experiencing, inwardly and outwardly. She saw that holding *whatever* was arising in nonjudgmental awareness was all that was required. It usually helped to broaden her field of awareness to include her body as a whole. This allowed Peggy both to see what was happening from moment to moment and to relate to her experience in a direct, nonconceptual way. She had found a different place to stand: behind the torrent of thoughts and feelings of the cascading mind. This was a little like standing behind a waterfall; she could move in close to it, seeing its force but not getting dragged along with it into the depths.

Adama's Story

Adama was 21 years old and came to mindfulness because she'd already been depressed twice during her teenage years, and didn't want to suffer her whole life. Now at college, she found that she could sometimes distract herself from her moods of despair, but there was so much to do, so many assignments to keep on top of, she began to get really afraid that she'd lose motivation and go back to how things had been in high school when she'd felt completely unable to cope. She had seen a therapist then, which had helped, but the depression felt like it was always close at hand, like a dark pit she might fall into at any time. Nights were the worst time, when there was nothing to distract her, and she couldn't so easily contact others. She would reach for her phone several times during a sleepless night, listen to a podcast, or swipe through TikTok videos. When she first tried mindfulness, she found it very challenging, as friends who'd told her about it said it would calm her mind, but it seemed to have the opposite effect.

"The hard part was realizing how much I've come to rely on my phone. I've never ever been without a phone, and whenever a gap appears in the day, I always reach for it to look to see whether I've got messages, to look for new Instagram posts, to check my BeReal contacts, as well as catching up with mail and listening to my playlists. It's my way of relaxing, as my downtime is always filled up with things I get from the phone. Then, in the pandemic, me and my classmates were totally dependent on our laptops and phones, because the teachers sent notifications about new assignments. The phone is my lifeline.

"When I started meditating at home, the silence was deafening. So, I was following the meditations on the phone, but there were all those gaps where it felt like nothing was happening. All that I could feel was an impulse to look at the phone to check for notifications! It was really bad in the first week. We were doing the body scan, and I saw how it might be relaxing if only I could focus more—and in the second week I found myself more relaxed than I had been for a long while. That felt a bit better.

"And then one day I was outside taking a break between lectures, sitting on a bench outside the lecture hall, and the sun came out, and I reached for my phone. As my hand reached for it, I stopped. I became aware that as I was reaching, something else was going on that I hadn't seen before. I sensed my body contract just for a moment—I felt a tension in my shoulders and a frown on my face. I saw that I'd been gearing up to see my messages, wondering if there'd be something funny, or some bad news, or another assignment, or just planning how to respond to what I found . . . the whole body was getting ready for doing something, even though I was thinking about relaxing. So I stopped reaching, then a space opened up around the tension. I felt the sun on my face and my feet on the ground, and my breath, and it was more than relaxation—it was a moment of pure joy."

Adama had discovered something that, in time, would shift her whole perspective about mindfulness practice and what it was like to inhabit an alternative, being mode of mind. Many people find meditation brings calm, and it's true that early on in MBCT, learning to anchor our wayward attention, and to focus in one place we have chosen, can feel grounding and relaxing. So it's easy to conclude that mindfulness is only about learning to attend in order to stabilize the mind and bring relaxation. Mindfulness does this, but it goes further: it builds on these early foundations to reveal new insights about the changeability of body sensations and thoughts and feelings and teaches us to see sensations, thoughts, feelings, and impulses as events in the body/mind coming and going, without taking them personally or judging ourselves harshly for having them. As we've seen in this book, our major ally in this is to learn to attend to the weather pattern in the body, this precious source of information that we easily ignore or suppress. The discovery that Adama made was important because, unbeknown to her, the body scan had been gradually allowing her to tune in to a source of information that she had little access to before.

"Listening to my body's signals—I didn't know what that even meant before. So now, when I use my phone, I'll count to three or take a couple of breaths each time I notice I'm reaching for it. In that moment I sense my body, and this gives me a heads-up about what I need right then—and I make a choice. Sometimes I do pick it up. Often I don't."

David's Story

From the moment he looked at the raisin during the first class, with its wrinkles, glistening highlights, and deep rich colors, David had become really enthusiastic about exploring mindfulness. The experience had reawakened in him memories of the times he had valued most in his life: times long ago when as a young man he sat on the dunes of a deserted beach, looking across a glistening sea to the horizon; or waking, fully refreshed, on a Sunday morning, drawing back the curtains to reveal an expanse of freshly fallen snow. These were times when he'd felt at one with the world, fully present and filled with gratitude for being alive.

For David, the realization that he could change his experience by changing the way he paid attention in each moment was immensely empowering. He threw himself into bringing mindfulness to each aspect of his day. Over time he learned to prioritize giving attention to physical sensations as a way to stay connected with the immediacy of his experience. As soon as he awoke, he took three deliberate, mindful breaths, sensing his abdomen rise and fall with each one, using the sensations in his body as a focus to gather his attention before it became entangled and dispersed in anticipating and planning the day ahead. In the shower, he used the first contact of the water as a reminder to enter fully into the present moment, to tune in to the sensations in his body—the tingling on his skin where the water splattered, the movements in his limbs as he rubbed soap over his body. As he dressed, he deliberately exaggerated the stretching and bending movements he made as he pulled on his shirt, tied his shoelaces, reminding himself to tune in to the sensations in his muscles, just as he had in practicing mindful yoga.

David changed the way he ate breakfast with the family. The TV no longer delivered the news, the disastrous state of the wider world and the local traffic, dimly attended in the background as the family got ready for the day. He no longer scrolled through the news apps on his phone, automatically placing food in his mouth, barely aware whether it was toast or cornflakes, coffee or tea, or which of the children it was who was shouting about not being able to find a bookbag. Now he held this time with greater awareness. He dedicated it to mindful presence: David's intention was to be here for these moments of his morning, for himself and for his family. After all, wasn't this his life?

David's way to work crossed some railroad tracks. Often the barriers would be down, blocking the way for cars, allowing a train to pass. In the past, he would respond with a sigh—"Oh God, not again!"—and sit there, hunched over the steering wheel. Now his response was "Okay, I've got an opportunity to do a breathing space here." He did as many of the three steps as time allowed—with his eyes open of course, to catch the time when the barrier lifted. Reconnected with the here and now, he put conscious effort into driving mindfully, attending to the sensations where his fingers touched the steering wheel, to the contact points of his body with the seat, and to the relevant sights through the windshield—the details of the other cars on the road, their colors, their patterns of movement. By the time he arrived in the parking lot at work, he no longer felt exhausted by the prospect of the day ahead.

Through his conscious efforts to be fully present in more of his moments, David had transformed and enriched the quality not only of his mornings, but also of his evenings and weekends. Family life became more of a pleasure than a burden once again. But what about the rest of his life, the bulk of his waking weekday hours that were spent at work?

Here the picture was not so simple. Much of David's work involved "being in his head"—thinking, planning, and writing reports, all under tight and pressing deadlines. Although he was much more ready to take on each day, David's attempts to bring mindfulness to these activities just "didn't seem to work"—it didn't seem possible to approach them in the same mindful way that he could approach eating his breakfast or listening to music or being with the family. He might begin his work with a clear intention to remain mindfully present, but within moments of sitting down to answer e-mails, write a report, or develop a plan or meeting agenda for his clients, he would "lose it"—he would get carried away, drawn into the task, the need to deliver an elegant solution, the need to look smart and avoid screwing up. Every now and then he would become aware of how much he had lost contact with the moment, but this would just make things worse—he would begin to feel disappointed, resentful of the way his work seemed to be robbing him of the possibilities for happiness and clarity that he had begun to experience in other areas of his life.

From time to time, it would occur to David to take a breathing space. Sometimes this was really helpful, allowing him to gather himself, regroup, and see more clearly what was going on. More often, he would emerge from Step 3 feeling that he still wasn't present with the spaciousness and clarity he was experiencing in other areas of his life. At such times, his main feeling was one of pressure to get back to the task at hand—to get the current assignment out of the way as quickly as possible, and *then* he could begin to explore how to be more mindful at work. But, of course, as soon as he finished one assignment, the next was sitting there waiting, calling for his attention. So he would immerse himself in that one to get it out of the way as soon as possible—*then* he might have the leisure to be mindful. But, like the end of the rainbow, that goal seemed to recede constantly despite his efforts to reach it.

For a while, David grudgingly resigned himself to the fact that work simply had to be endured; his workplace seemed a no-go area as far as mindfulness was concerned. So he decided to put his energies into being mindful before and after work and to "shut down" while he was there, to just plow ahead with what needed to get done. But the sense that something was awry would not go away. He began to fantasize about giving up his job, moving the family to the country and living a simple life, growing their own food, tending a few animals, perhaps becoming a potter. He wondered about working even harder and longer for a few years, so that he could save enough to give it all up.

Fortunately, David continued to practice mindfulness and also to explore it more through reading books on meditation, listening to podcasts, and attending live talks by meditation teachers. Together with his own practice, this immersion led over time to a shift in David's approach. He became aware that he was not alone in the kind of problems he faced— even famous meditation teachers did not find it easy to bring mindfulness to work that involved a lot of "head" tasks! Thich Nhat Hanh, a renowned and highly respected Vietnamese meditation teacher who introduced thousands in the West to mindfulness through his numerous books and retreats, said at one point that he found it possible to be mindful when binding books by hand, but difficult when writing them. David found this admission enormously liberating. The fact that he found it difficult to combine mindfulness with "head" tasks didn't mean something was wrong with him. It was an inherent aspect of this kind of task that it was difficult to sustain awareness. Another well-known teacher described how he would shift mental mode by tuning in to sensory awareness for a minute or two at least once every half hour while writing or working on other "head" tasks: he might go outside for a mindful walk or stroll, feeling the movements of his body, the coolness of the fresh air on his face, hearing the sounds of the birds. In this way he was checking in,

> **Breaking up "head" tasks periodically and widening our awareness to the world around us can keep us from slipping too far away from being mode.**

however briefly, to being mode, reconnecting with that mode so that it never slipped far away.

Inspired in this way, David renewed his intention to bring mindfulness, as best he could, into his work situation. He found it a great relief to acknowledge explicitly the difficulty of what he was trying to do, rather than feeling that it was something he "should" have been able to do and feeling like a failure. He also found some benefit from the "mode breaks," which for him often took the form of standing upright, gently stretching, focusing on his breathing, on the sensations in the soles of his feet where he could feel grounded, connected to the earth below, and on physical sensations throughout his body as he gently stretched upward. But he still found himself making negative comparisons with the levels of presence and clarity that he was able to sustain outside work—he still felt a long way away from that kind of mindfulness.

And then, at one point, he happened to take another look at meditation teacher Larry Rosenberg's guidelines for mindful living:

Five steps for practicing mindfulness throughout the day:

1. When possible, do just one thing at a time.
2. Pay full attention to what you are doing.
3. When the mind wanders from what you are doing, bring it back.
4. Repeat step number three several billion times.
5. Investigate your distractions.

David had found Steps 1–4 invaluable guides to being more mindful in his wider life; he especially appreciated the wisdom and humor of Step 4. But he had never really gotten into Step 5, and, in fact, was not really sure what it meant. So he decided that it might be good to include some breathing spaces—after all, the instructions for Step 1 of the breathing space invited him to *become aware* of what was going on in his experience: thoughts, feelings, bodily sensations. Up to this point he had treated this step very cursorily, giving a brief nod of acknowledgment to his experience before passing on to, as he saw it, the real business of Steps 2 and 3. So now he lingered longer over Step 1, intentionally looking a little more closely at what thoughts, feelings, and physical sensations he was experiencing each time he took a "mode break" at work. And he was shocked by what he found: the extent of the unhappiness, discontent, and longing in his feelings; the number of times his thoughts revolved around "I don't want this—I want that"; the levels of tension, resistance, and aversion he discovered in his body. David was appalled. But he was also aware of the beginnings of a sense of compassion for the pain that he now recognized.

As he persisted with his exploratory breathing spaces, David became increasingly aware that his doing mind was very busy. What was it up to? It was busy doing what it was always doing: computing the match or mismatch—the size of the gap—between goals and the current state of affairs. For David, operating in doing mode meant that, in the background, his mind was comparing the state in which he found himself at work with the mindful, clear, peaceful state that he longed for, creating further unhappiness in the process. It came to him that what he was experiencing was "craving"—a longing for things to be other than they are. Over and over again, he became aware of just how unhappy this was making him. Eventually, he knew deep in his bones, not just in his head, that he was creating this suffering himself. And, with that insight came a compassionate response: Why not do yourself a favor and let go? The words *"I do not need to be happy"* came to him. As he said these words to himself, David experienced a wonderful sense of lightness come over him, as if a burden that he had been carrying for too long had suddenly been lifted from him. And he felt happy!

> Letting go of happiness as a goal can pave the way for happiness to appear on its own.

David continues to work at the same job—he still does not experience the same clarity and peace there that he knows is available to him in his wider life, but he can sit more lightly with his work situation. He is able to respond with more kindness and compassion, to take better care of himself in this difficult setting. He knows now, deep down, that mindfulness is much more than paying closer attention to the color of the trees or the sounds of the birds, delightful as these are. He knows that mindfulness also provides a way to discern those patterns of mind that serve us and those patterns of mind that create and perpetuate suffering. And he has discovered what each of us may discover in our own way: that we have a source of profound wisdom within our own minds and bodies and hearts.

EVERYDAY MINDFULNESS

Here are some tips that many in our mindfulness classes have found helpful:

■ When you first wake up in the morning before you get out of bed, bring your attention to your breathing for at least five full breaths, letting the breath "breathe itself."

■ Notice your body posture. Be aware of how your body and mind feel when you move from lying down to sitting, to standing, to walking. Notice each time you make a transition from one posture to the next.

■ When you hear a phone ring, a bird sing, a train pass by, laughter, a car horn, the wind, or the sound of a door closing, use it or any other sound to remind you to come fully into the here and now. Really listen, being present and awake.

■ Throughout the day, take a few moments to bring your attention to your breathing for at least five full breaths.

■ When you eat or drink something, take a minute and breathe. Bring awareness to seeing your food, smelling your food, tasting your food, chewing your food, and swallowing your food.

■ When you find yourself reaching for your phone, take a deliberate pause for at least one in-breath and out-breath and make a choice about whether or not to check it.

■ Notice your body while walking or standing. Take a moment to notice your posture. Pay attention to the contact of the ground under your feet. Feel the air on your face, arms, and legs as you walk. Are you rushing to get to the next moment? Even when you are in a hurry, *be with* the hurrying; check in with yourself to see whether you are "making extra" by telling yourself all the things that might go wrong.

■ Bring awareness to listening and talking. Can you listen without having to agree or disagree, fall into liking or disliking, or planning what you will say when it's your turn? Can you just say what you need to say without overstating or understating it? Can you notice how your mind and body feel? Can you notice what is conveyed by your tone of voice? Is your speaking an improvement on silence?

▪ When you find yourself waiting in a line, use this time to notice standing and breathing. Feel the contact of your feet on the floor and how your body feels. Bring attention to the rising and falling of your abdomen. Are you feeling impatient?

▪ Be aware of any points of tightness in your body throughout the day. See if you can breathe into them, and as you exhale, let go of any excess tension. Be aware of any tension stored in your body. Is there tension in your neck, your shoulders, or in the stomach, the jaw, or your lower back? Get to know your aversion patterns (see Chapter 7). If possible, stretch or do yoga once a day.

▪ Focus attention on your daily activities—such as brushing your teeth, brushing your hair, washing up, or putting on your shoes. Bring mindfulness to each activity.

▪ Before you go to sleep at night, take a few minutes and bring your attention to your breathing for at least five full breaths.

▪ If you wish to maintain a daily practice and aren't sure what to do, then you might go through the week-by-week program included here, but taking a month over each step rather than a week. Practicing the same set of meditations for a whole month (or even longer) can reveal more of their potential, and allow you to discover a profound kindness toward yourself, just as you are.

Becoming Fully Alive

It is not that difficult situations, worries, memories, or people are somehow neutralized by our practice of mindfulness or that we become indifferent to them. Rather, the space we make for them when we bring present-moment awareness to them is bigger; it is big enough for them to become only part of our experience. We may find ourselves starting to make more room in the present moment for realizing and embodying the full spectrum of who we already are, wherever we are. We may come to trust ourselves in new and different ways. We may discover that we are okay as we are and that we can accept ourselves as we are. We may begin to feel a growing sense of gratitude for the life we already have, rather than grasping at the one we fantasize about. We may decide to accept the chance to see and to savor the wonders of the life available to us, as our life is unfolding moment by moment. This is the great adventure of mindfulness, the great adventure of being alive.

When our minds are incessantly preoccupied with the rewards or dangers that may await us at the end of our journey, we are cutting ourselves off from the richness of life itself, and from our ability to recognize it in the texture of each moment along the way. In any one moment, this may seem no great loss—but a whole life of lost moments is a whole life lost.

LOVE AFTER LOVE

The time will come
when, with elation,
you will greet yourself arriving
at your own door, in your own mirror,
and each will smile at the other's welcome

and say, sit here. Eat.
You will love again the stranger who was your self.
Give wine. Give bread. Give back your heart
to itself, to the stranger who has loved you

all your life, whom you have ignored
for another, who knows you by heart.
Take down the love letters from the bookshelf,

the photographs, the desperate notes,
peel your own image from the mirror.
Sit. Feast on your life.

—DEREK WALCOTT, *The Poetry of Derek Walcott 1948–2013*

The tragedy for too many of us is not that our lives are too short, but that we take so long before we start to live them. The source of wisdom we discover from the practice of mindfulness, if we allow it, will eventually show us the immense and tragic suffering that stems from unawareness. It will allow us to see, to dwell in, and to treasure the deep peace that lies at the heart of each moment if we have the courage to cultivate awareness, here and now. It will allow us to experience being fully alive—here and now, while we have the chance.

Eleven

Bringing It All Together

WEAVING THE MINDFULNESS
PROGRAM INTO YOUR LIFE

Whether or not you've been sampling the practices in this book as you have been going along, perhaps you are now drawn to systematically engage in and experience the whole program for yourself. In this chapter we take you step by step through the eight-session mindfulness-based cognitive therapy for depression program. The best way to approach this work is to set aside an eight-week period in which you can commit to spending an

---

LOOKING AFTER YOURSELF

If you are experiencing an episode of depression right now, then take things step by step. Recent research shows that MBCT can be helpful in these circumstances, but if things are really bad right now, and your depression makes it just too difficult to concentrate on some of the practices, it might be most skillful to allow yourself to wait a while if you can, as it can be disheartening to struggle with new learning when you are feeling overwhelmed. If you do start, remember that it is fine to take a break for a while and return to it when you feel that you have the resources, that you are not too upset, nor too tired. So, be very gentle with yourself—remembering that the difficulties you experience are a direct effect of depression and will, sooner or later, ease.

---

hour each day engaging in the various meditation practices and exercises outlined here.

As with acquiring any new skill, engaging in the mindfulness practices described here will involve something of a shift in how we approach learning. Take swimming as an example. There comes a point when the teacher has to stop telling us how and invite us into the water. *Describing* how to stay afloat, no matter how good the description, is simply not enough; we need to *experience* it for ourselves, directly. The same is true for mindfulness practice. As with swimming, it can feel a bit intimidating to make the transition from talking about it to actually experiencing it firsthand (especially for those of us who have gotten used to being pretty competent in other areas of life). In both cases, some persistence in practice will be required. A short dip in the water will not be enough to learn to swim. Similarly, a session or two dipping into meditation may not be that useful in the long term. Mindfulness meditation can feel exciting and illuminating at times, but it can also feel downright boring, especially in the early stages, until we learn how to work with mind states and feeling states such as boredom. At different times, we certainly will encounter restlessness, frustration, and impatience, as well as many other mind states and body states. That is not a problem at all, as long as we remember that it is possible to hold it all lightly in awareness in any moment. Week by week, we introduce new elements to the daily practice, so that over the eight weeks you will be continually building on, as well as deepening, what you've already learned. It's important to take your time with the meditation practices. Follow along with the instructions on the audio-guidance tracks as best you can, even if it feels difficult, boring, or repetitive at times. If something feels difficult, our outcome-oriented doing-obsessed minds may be tempted to rush on to the next practice, hoping to find something more peaceful. Instead, see if you can remember that the intention is not to strive for some goal, not even to be relaxed or to find peace of mind. Pleasant feelings, if they arise in some moments, are a welcome by-product of the practice, but they are by no means "the" goal of the practice. If there is any "goal," it is merely that of being fully present with openhearted spaciousness with whatever arises in experience, to be awake, to be fully alive, to be fully who we already are at our core.

There is no question that effort is required in the practice of meditation, but it is the wise effort of patience, commitment, and trust rather than the effort of continually checking to see how much "progress" you've made toward what you think is your "destination." It is rather like hoping that a butterfly will settle on your shoulder. Trying to make it do so and getting more and more agitated if it doesn't only makes it less likely to happen. In the end, you just have to give up trying and see if the butterfly lands by itself.

It is wise to put time aside on a daily basis for the more formal cultivation of mindfulness using the various practices described in the book. Try to view this time as a special time for yourself, and so protect and respect it accordingly. It is not selfish to take such time for ourselves. On the contrary, it is an act of wisdom and self-compassion to take such time for dropping in on the present moment, whatever we find here. Dedicating a specific place and a particular time in which to practice may mean rearranging your life a bit. Few of us have a spare hour in each day that is not already accounted for by family or work commitments—or sleep. So, for eight weeks, some of these commitments may have to be modified or rearranged. It can be challenging in some ways to do this, even for two months, but it's essential to make such a commitment and then stick with it through thick and thin, as part of the discipline inherent in mindfulness. Otherwise, our worthy intention to practice will inevitably get squeezed out by other, seemingly higher, priorities. The doing mind will always be more than happy to present a compelling case for not practicing "today" or for cutting corners on our commitment. You may find it most effective to wake up earlier in the morning and devote that time to formal practice. If so, perhaps you will need to go to bed earlier so that your practice is not done entirely at the expense of needed sleep. When you have settled on a time and a place, it is best to make arrangements so that you will be warm and comfortable, telling whoever needs to know what you are up to so that you will not be disturbed or interrupted. Switch your phone to airplane mode if possible, or, if a call or notification does come through during the time you have set aside for practicing, see if it is possible to let it be, being "out" for whoever is calling or messaging and "in" for yourself. That alone is a powerful and nurturing practice, a small antidote to 24/7 connectivity. We can look at this time as a time to connect with ourselves for a change, an increasingly rare event for all of us.

While we occasionally have to deal with external interruptions of our practice, it is the internal "interruptions" that are the most challenging. For indeed, we are continually interrupting ourselves. This becomes very apparent when we begin to observe the activity of our own minds as we attempt to maintain a particular focus of attention. Those interruptions can take many different forms, such as the wandering mind, the wanting mind, the judging mind, the planning mind, the worrying mind, and the obsessing, ruminating mind. We will be constantly visited by thoughts of things we just remembered we need to do and the accompanying feeling of having to "act right now." If this happens, see if you can experiment with letting all these ideas and plans, judgments, and self-talk come and go in your mind like clouds in the sky, rather than reacting to them as if you had to go and do whatever it is right now. And let's refrain as best we can from turning the meditation practice into one more "thing" we now have to *do*. For it is not a doing, it is simply being, and being yourself.

When we are guiding groups of patients through an eight-week mindfulness program, we find it essential, before each session, to remind ourselves of our own intentions and larger "agenda" for that session. In the same spirit, we recommend that you begin each week by reviewing the relevant chapters of this book. To help you do this, we highlight them at the beginning of the suggested program outlined here for each of the eight weeks. That would be a good time to incorporate the additional exercises described in each chapter, if you have not already done so.

Last, it is important to remember that you don't have to find the practice enjoyable. In fact, you don't have to like it at all. The challenge is just to take it on for eight weeks, following the instructions in as wholehearted a way as you can manage, suspending judgment along the way. As best you can, let go of all agendas, even to get better, and see what happens, moment by moment, day by day, and week by week. Keep to the practices day by day with the intention that this discipline, this radical act of being with yourself, of taking time for yourself, will become an intimate part of your life, part of your daily routine, but without ever becoming routine. The invitation is to always be opening to the new, because each moment is new, and unique, and available to us.

On this adventure of dropping in on ourselves and recognizing how fully alive we are or can be, we are responsible only for what we bring to the practice, the input. The output, or outcome, is predictable in some ways, and in other ways it is completely unpredictable. Any outcomes will be unique for each of us and continually changing anyway. None of us can tell in advance what is to be discovered in some future present moment. All we get to work with is now. If we can be here for this moment of now, with things exactly as they already are, that is the practice. The rest takes care of itself.

The second most important thing to remember is to practice every day even if, on some days, it might be for only five minutes. The *most* important thing is to remember that the real practice is none other than your life.

Week 1 (Chapters 3 and 5)

For the first week of your formal practice, we recommend that you do the *body scan*, using the instructions on Track 2 of the audio files that accompany this book. Do it every day, whether you feel like it or not. You will have to experiment with what the best time of day is for you to practice, but remember, the idea is to "fall awake," not to fall asleep. If you have a lot of trouble with sleepiness, try practicing with your eyes open or sitting up.

To cultivate mindfulness in your daily life—what we have been calling "informal practice"—you might try bringing moment-to-moment awareness to routine activities such as brushing your teeth, showering, drying your body, getting dressed, eating, driving, or taking out the garbage. The list of possibilities is endless, but the point is simply to zero-in on *knowing what you are doing as you are actually doing it* and on what you are thinking and feeling from moment to moment as well. You may find it helpful just to pick out one routine activity each week, such as brushing your teeth, and see if you can remember to be fully with the activity when you do it, every time you do it, as best you can. Of course, this is not so easy, so forgetting and then remembering again also becomes an important part of this practice. In addition, you might try to eat at least one meal during the week mindfully.

Week 2 (Chapter 4)

Continue practicing the *body scan* each day, guided by the instructions on Track 2 of the audio files. You may find it helpful to remember that the body scan is a foundational practice, the virtues of which may not be apparent for some time. In addition to the body scan, practice *mindfulness of breathing* while sitting for ten minutes (Track 4) at some other time during the day.

For informal practice in Week 2, we suggest you extend your mindfulness of everyday activities by adding a new routine activity that you carry out each day, and make a particular point of being present and attentive for this activity, as well as the one you chose for Week 1. It would also be a good idea to try to be aware of *one pleasant event* per day in your life *as it is happening.* Keep a calendar for the week, jotting down what the experience was, whether you were actually aware of it at the time it was happening (that's the assignment, but it doesn't always work out that way), how your body felt at the time, what thoughts and feelings were present, and what thoughts pass through your mind at the time you are writing it down. A sample calendar is provided on pages 232–233.

Week 3 (Chapters 6 and 9)

We recommend that in Week 3 you stop doing the body scan for a while and replace it with longer daily sittings, each preceded by ten minutes of gentle, mindful yoga. You may find that the simplest way to do this is, first, to make sure that the place you sit will be ready and then go right through the instructions on Tracks 3 (*mindful standing yoga*), 4 (*mindfulness of the breath*), and 5 (*mindfulness of the breath and body*). If you wish to explore the mindful yoga more deeply as part of your practice, you can find longer guided mindful yoga sequences that we use in our MBSR programs as part of the Series 1 Guided Mindfulness Meditation Practice Programs with Jon Kabat-Zinn, obtainable online from *www.jonkabat-zinn.com.* A mindful yoga meditation guided by Zindel Segal and used as part of our MBCT classes is also available on Track 9. Remember to do in the yoga only what you feel your body is capable of and always to err on the side of being conservative, listening carefully to your body's messages as you practice. Remember also to check with your doctor or physical therapist if you have chronic pain, any kind of musculoskeletal problem, or lung or heart disease.

Week 3 is a good time to begin practicing the *three-minute breathing space* (Chapter 9). We suggest you begin by doing it three times a day at set

PRACTICE AT A GLANCE FOR THE EIGHT-WEEK MINDFULNESS PROGRAM

Week	Daily practice
1	Body scan (Track 2) Mindfulness in daily living
2	Body scan (Track 2) Pleasant Events Calendar (pages 232–233) Ten-minute sitting with awareness of breath (Track 4)
3	Mindful standing yoga, breath, and body (Tracks 3, 4, and 5) Yoga (see text, page 230) Unpleasant Events Calendar (pages 235–236) Three-minute breathing space (Track 7)
4	Mindful standing yoga, breath, and body (Tracks 3, 4, and 5) Awareness of pleasant/unpleasant feelings Three-minute breathing space (Track 7)
5	Mindfulness of breath and body, then exploring a difficulty (Track 10) Three-minute breathing space (Track 7), opening the body door (pages 193–196)
6	Mindfulness of breath, body, sounds, thoughts, and choiceless awareness (Tracks 4, 5, and 6 or Track 11) Three-minute breathing space (Track 7), opening the thought door (pages 196–198)
7	Alternate daily (1) meditation of choice (without audio recording; forty minutes per day) with (2) mindfulness of breath, body, sounds, thoughts, and choiceless awareness (Track 11) Three-minute breathing space (Track 7), opening the door of skillful action (pages 198–201)
8	The rest of your life: choose a sustainable pattern of formal and informal mindfulness practice

Pleasant Events Calendar

Be aware of a pleasant event at the time it is happening. Use these questions to focus your awareness on the details of the experience as it is happening. Write it down as soon as possible afterward.

	What was the experience?	How did your body feel, in detail, during this experience?	What thoughts or images accompanied this event? (write thoughts in words; describe images)	What moods, feelings, and emotions accompanied this event?	What thoughts are in your mind now as you write this down?
Example:	Heading home at the end of my shift—stopping, hearing a bird sing	Lightness across the face, aware of shoulders dropping, uplift of corners of mouth	"That's good," "How lovely" (the bird), "It's so nice to be outside."	Relief, pleasure	"It was such a small thing, but I'm glad I noticed it."
Monday					
Tuesday					
Wednesday					

(continued)

What was the experience?	How did your body feel, in detail, during this experience?	What thoughts or images accompanied this event? (write thoughts in words; describe images)	What moods, feelings, and emotions accompanied this event?	What thoughts are in your mind now as you write this down?
Thursday				
Friday				
Saturday				
Sunday				

times that you have decided on in advance. Use the instructions on Track 7 for guidance until you get the hang of it and then practice giving yourself the instructions in the same way.

For informal practice in Week 3, try to be aware, in detail, of your experience of *one unpleasant or stressful event* each day. Observe and record these unpleasant events in just the same way that you did with the pleasant events in Week 2. A sample calendar is provided on pages 235–236.

Week 4 (Chapter 6)

For daily formal practice in Week 4, we suggest that you continue with the sequence of *mindful standing yoga* (Track 3), *mindfulness of the breath* (Track 4), and *mindfulness of the breath and body* (Track 5). This week, see if you can use this practice as a time to tune in especially to feelings of pleasantness and unpleasantness (Chapter 6) from moment to moment. If you become aware of any experiences that are particularly intense or unpleasant, or of any strong feelings of aversion or disliking while you are practicing, you might try using these as opportunities to experiment with *responding* more skillfully and gently to what is difficult and unwanted as opposed to merely *reacting*.

Continue to take a *breathing space* three times every day, at regular times that you have scheduled in advance. In addition, you might like to begin to experiment with intentionally responding to the unpleasant and stressful events in your day-to-day life. Do this by taking a three-minute breathing space whenever you become aware that you are having difficulty remaining present or when you feel unhappy, stressed, or thrown off balance.

Week 5 (Chapter 7)

In Week 5 we suspend the mindful yoga, although, of course, you can always continue it if you care to. However, the primary focus of the formal practice this week is becoming more aware of aversion and cultivating gentle ways of responding to unpleasant feelings with greater allowing and acceptance. You have a choice here: you can start with the *mindfulness of the breath, and*

Unpleasant Events Calendar

Be aware of an unpleasant event at the time it is happening. Use these questions to focus your awareness on the details of the experience as it is happening. Write it down as soon as possible afterward.

What was the experience?	How did your body feel, in detail, during this experience?	What thoughts or images accompanied this event? (write thoughts in words; describe images)	What moods, feelings, and emotions accompanied this event?	What thoughts are in your mind now as you write this down?
Example: Waiting in line at the store and someone pushes ahead of me	Tightness around my eyes, my jaw was clenched, then my shoulders sort of slumped	"I should be firm," "some people only look after themselves," "If I weren't so invisible, people wouldn't push me around."	I felt angry and taken advantage of. Then I felt guilty for not standing up myself.	"If something seems unfair, I always blame myself."
Monday				
Tuesday				
Wednesday				

(continued)

235

What was the experience?	How did your body feel, in detail, during this experience?	What thoughts or images accompanied this event? (write thoughts in words; describe images)	What moods, feelings, and emotions accompanied this event?	What thoughts are in your mind now as you write this down?
Thursday				
Friday				
Saturday				
Sunday				

of the breath and body, using the instructions on Tracks 4 and 5, and then turning off the audio and continuing by yourself by deliberately allowing a difficulty or concern to come to mind (as described on pages 150–151). Or, if you wish to follow a complete audio-guidance track for exploring difficulty (including mindfulness of breath and body), you can use Track 10.

If you choose to work on your own to explore difficulty, use the suggestions given in Chapter 7 to experiment with different ways to respond more gently and kindly to unpleasant feelings and body sensations. Throughout these explorations, be sure to take good care of yourself, using the guidelines in Chapter 7. After being with a difficulty or concern for five minutes or so in this way, you may find it helpful to conclude your daily sitting with a three-minute breathing space (Track 7).

As in Week 4, continue to do a *three-minute breathing space* three times a day at your regular scheduled times and also whenever you become aware of unpleasant feelings. This week you might like to explore the option of opening the body door (Chapter 9, pages 193–196).

Week 6 (Chapter 8)

In Week 6, the focus is on thinking. For your daily formal practice we recommend running through the sequence of Tracks 4 (*mindfulness of the breath*), 5 (*mindfulness of breath and body*), and 6 (*mindfulness of sounds and thoughts*). Toward the end of the instructions on Track 6 (*mindfulness of sounds and thoughts*), you will find instructions for cultivating *choiceless awareness*. We suggest that you shut off the audio guidance after this track and continue on your own in silence for a period of time, using the instructions at the end of that track and also the instructions outlined in Chapter 8 (page 176). Then you might find it useful to finish off with a three-minute breathing space (Track 7). If you wish to follow a complete audio-guidance track for mindfulness of breath, body, sounds, thoughts, and choiceless awareness, you can use Track 11, narrated by John Teasdale.

Continue to use the *breathing space* three times a day at previously scheduled times and whenever you experience unpleasant feelings. This week you might like to focus particularly on the thoughts that are present in those moments in which you experience unpleasant feelings. One way to do this is to follow the practice we call opening the thought door (Chapter 9, pages 196–198).

By this time you will probably want to be making the decisions for yourself about when and what to practice and for how long. After four or five weeks, many people feel ready to start crafting and personalizing their own meditation practice more and more, using our guidelines merely as suggestions. By the end of the eight weeks our aim is for you to have made the practice your own by adapting it to suit your schedule, your needs, and your temperament in terms of which combination of formal and informal techniques you find most helpful.

Week 7 (Chapters 3 and 9)

To encourage self-directed practice, alternate days this week are dedicated to practicing without the audio guidance, if at all possible. We recommend that, on these days, you devote a total of forty minutes per day to a combination of sitting, mindful yoga, and the body scan, deciding on the mix yourself. We encourage you to experiment, perhaps using two or even three of the practices on the same day. On one day you might do yoga for ten minutes, followed by twenty minutes of sitting meditation right after it, with perhaps a ten-minute body scan at another time of day entirely. On another day, having spent ten minutes practicing mindfulness of the breath, you might continue sitting with choiceless awareness for the rest of the forty minutes.

On the alternate days, we recommend using the suggestions for formal practice given for Week 6 (Tracks 4, 5, and 6), followed by continuing with optional choiceless awareness (page 176), or just returning to an awareness of the breath. Track 11 offers this sequence in one sitting meditation if you prefer.

At this point, you may find it helpful to reflect on your practice of the three-minute breathing space by rereading Chapter 9. Continue with the regular, scheduled, breathing spaces three times a day. When responding to unpleasant events with a breathing space, focus this week on the option of opening the door of skillful action (Chapter 9, pages 198–201).

Week 8 (Chapter 10)

Week 8 in the program is the time to decide what, for you, will be the pattern of daily mindfulness practice that you will settle into for the future if you decide that the practice of mindfulness is valuable enough for you to keep nurturing it. This is a good time to revisit all the formal practices, including the body scan, by working your way through Tracks 2 through 11 of the audio guidance in whatever order and combination you choose. The pattern of practice that you finally choose might, of course, be based on taking yourself through one or more of these practices without using any guidance at all. In our experience, almost without exception, people have found it invaluable to include the breathing space as part of their daily practice. In Chapter 10 ("Everyday Mindfulness" box, pages 221–222) you will find more suggestions for how to keep up the momentum of mindfulness practice and deepen it over the years.

The eighth week is the end of our formal recommendations for practice, but it also marks the first week of practicing entirely on your own. We tell participants in our classes that the eighth week really represents the rest of your life. It is a new beginning as much as it is a noteworthy completion, not really an end of anything. Life keeps unfolding, the breath keeps unfolding, our moments keep unfolding. The practice doesn't end just because we have reached this point in our journey together. By now you will be firmly in the driver's seat yourself in one manner of speaking and probably feeling like an utter novice at the same time, left to your own devices far too prematurely. This is a totally natural feeling. It is also based on reality, as the practice of mindfulness is really endless, as is the potential for each of us to grow into ourselves. But if, up to this point, you have been able to practice in a regular, disciplined way, as we have been encouraging you to do, chances are you will have tasted enough of the abundance of the present moment to want to continue to inhabit your life in a way that honors being and lets whatever doing we engage in, inwardly and outwardly, to flow out of our being. By this point, whether the thinking, judging mind believes it or not, you will have developed enough skill and experience to keep up the momentum you have generated through your own efforts over these eight weeks. And this momentum, coupled with the inherent wisdom of your own heart, will continue to guide and shape the deepening of your own mindfulness practice and help you to embrace fully, through thick and thin, this ongoing adventure we call life.

All contemporary meditation teachers, ourselves included, encourage students to carve out time from their busy lives to do some kind of formal meditation practice every day, such as sitting quietly, aware of the breath breathing itself. It does not matter how long we give to the practice; all that matters is that we make the attempt to pause within all the doing and moving forward and practice, however brief it is by the clock, on a daily basis. Ultimately, mindfulness is not about time; it is about now. So even brief moments by the clock, if we are really present for them with awareness, in being mode, are profoundly reorienting and healing. However, to really know the landscape of our own mind and body, it is important to visit on a regular basis, or perhaps take up permanent residency, so to speak, rather than being a perpetual tourist. It may even be important, sooner or later, to learn the language. As with gaining fluency in a foreign language, living immersed in it and making use of it over and over again become extremely important. Fluency is kept alive through regular practice.

If you cultivate mindfulness on a regular basis, you almost can't help discovering that your mind has deep inner resources you hardly knew existed. Or even if you suspected as much, you probably didn't know that they could be systematically accessed from the depths of your own mind and heart and body and put to wise use for both your own benefit and the well-being of others. You may find yourself suddenly surprised to discover life situations in which a fresh and clearer perspective on things arises spontaneously and unbidden. You may be astonished when it takes the form of a spaciousness in your heart and mind that carries with it a sense of being free—free to be in wiser relationship to whatever is unfolding and also to be able to let go when appropriate and move on in ways that had before seemed impossible, even inconceivable. You are discovering an inner wisdom within yourself, a wisdom that can transform your emotions and your life. Once you have tasted this for yourself and seen the possibility of drinking even more deeply at this well, nothing can ever be quite the same again.

Notes

INTRODUCTION: Tired of Feeling So Bad for So Long

PAGE 1

Depression hurts: Many authors have explored depression from their own experience in ways that are helpful for others. The descriptions of depression and other mood problems in this paragraph come from the following: Jamison, K. R. (1995). *An unquiet mind.* New York: Knopf; Solomon, A. (2001). *The noonday demon.* New York: Scribner; Styron, W. (1994). *Darkness visible.* New York: Random House.

PAGE 3

Comprehensive reviews of data: Kuyken and colleagues' 2016 meta-analysis examined outcomes from 1,258 patients from nine clinical trials conducted worldwide. Kuyken, W., Warren, F., Taylor, R., et al. (2016). Efficacy of mindfulness-based cognitive therapy in prevention of depressive relapse: An individual patient data meta-analysis from randomized trials. *JAMA Psychiatry, 73*(6), 565–574.

reduction in risk of relapse: Patients with recurrent depression who experienced maltreatment in childhood were at lower risk of relapse following MBCT compared to those without early trauma. Williams, M., Crane, C., Barnhofer, T., et al. (2014). Mindfulness-based cognitive therapy for preventing relapse in recurrent depression: A randomized dismantling trial. *Journal of Consulting and Clinical Psychology, 82*(2), 275–286.

maintaining sensory awareness: Farb and colleagues tracked the brain activity of 85 formerly depressed patients as they watched sad and neutral film clips and were then followed for a period of 24 months. Participants at highest risk of relapse were the ones whose sensory cortices showed less activity while watching the sad film clips, compared to the neutral clips. In fact, sensory shutdown was associated with an eightfold increase in the emergence of a new episode of depression over the follow up. Farb, N., Desormeau, P., Anderson, A., et al. (2022). Static and treatment-responsive brain biomarkers of depression relapse vulnerability following prophylactic psychotherapy: Evidence from a randomized control trial. *NeuroImage: Clinical, 34*, 102969.

PAGE 5

enormously empowering for patients: Mindfulness-based interventions for a variety of health conditions were found to be similar to specific active controls and evidence-based treatments. Goldberg, S., Riordan, K., Sun, S., et al. (2022). The empirical status of mindfulness-based interventions: A systematic review of 44 meta-analyses of randomized controlled trials. *Perspectives on Psychological Science, 7*(1), 108–130.

These benefits have been confirmed: Mindfulness meditation emphasizes a different approach to negative affect and its neural signature. Farb, N., Anderson, A., Mayberg, H., et al. (2010). Minding one's emotions: Mindfulness training alters the neural expression of sadness. *Emotion, 10*(1), 25–33.

PAGE 6

MBCT manual: Segal, Z. V., Williams, J. M. G., & Teasdale, J. D. (2013). *Mindfulness-based cognitive therapy for depression, second edition.* New York: Guilford Press.

MBCT has taken its place: MBCT is included in an updated and expanded meta-analysis of psychological prophylaxis for depression. Breedvelt, J., Karyotaki, E., Warren, F., et al. (2024). An individual participant data meta-analysis of psychological interventions for preventing depression relapse. *Nature Mental Health, 2,* 154–163.

more effective than self-help cognitive therapy: The reliance on *The Mindful Way Workbook* for treatment delivery provides a scalable approach for increasing access to care. Strauss, C., Bibby-Jones, A., Jones, F., et al. (2023). Clinical effectiveness and cost-effectiveness of supported mindfulness-based cognitive therapy self-help compared with supported cognitive behavioral therapy self-help for adults experiencing depression: The low-intensity guided help through mindfulness (LIGHT-Mind) randomized clinical trial. *JAMA Psychiatry, 80*(5), 415–424.

adopted in health systems: MBCT is now one of the recommended interventions in many current international clinical guidelines including the United States (2019), Canada (2016), England (2009 and 2019 updated draft NICE depression guideline), Scotland (2010), and Wales (2016).

PAGE 7

MBCT in these "routine clinical practice" settings: Community-based data on MBCT's effectiveness is especially important in light of the fact that initial efficacy data were collected almost entirely in academic hospital settings. Tickell, A., Ball, S., Bernard, P., et al. (2020). The effectiveness of mindfulness-based cognitive therapy (MBCT) in real-world healthcare services. *Mindfulness, 11*(2), 279–290.

training to parliamentarians and staff: In the United Kingdom, an All-Party Parliamentary Group (APPG) on Mindfulness was established in 2014, and it commissioned the first *U.K. Mindful Nation Report* (see *www.themindfulnessinitiative.org*), followed by international political engagement and dissemination of the model of MBCT used in the U.K. parliament to thirty-nine other countries. See Ruane, C.

(2021). "Be the change you want to see": A politician's perspective on mindfulness in politics. *The Humanistic Psychologist, 49,* 56–71.

reducing current depression: Some early evidence suggests MBCT can offer relief to people who are in the midst of a major depressive episode. Strauss, C., Cavanagh, K., Oliver, A., et al. (2014). Mindfulness-based interventions for people diagnosed with a current episode of an anxiety or depressive disorder: A meta-analysis of randomised controlled trials. *PLOS One, 9*(4), e96110.

delivered by online therapy systems: A digitally delivered version of MBCT—Mindful Mood Balance—when added to treatment as usual for depression, was associated with more rapid reduction in residual depressive symptoms compared to usual care alone. Segal, Z., Dimidjian, S., Beck, A., et al. (2020). Outcomes of online mindfulness-based cognitive therapy for patients with residual depressive symptoms: A randomized clinical trial. *JAMA Psychiatry, 77*(6), 563–573.

meditation practice in the program: Meta-analysis reveals a small but significant effect size supporting the association between frequency of home practice and clinical outcomes. Parsons, C., Crane, C., Parsons, L., et al. (2017). Home practice in mindfulness-based cognitive therapy and mindfulness-based stress reduction: A systematic review and meta-analysis of participants' mindfulness practice and its association with outcomes. *Behaviour Research and Therapy, 95,* 29–41.

PAGE 8

MBCT increases mental flexibility: The ability to pause automatic routines and consider alternatives is a hallmark of effective emotion regulation. Greenberg, J., Reiner, K., & Meiran, N. (2012). "Mind the trap": Mindfulness practice reduces cognitive rigidity. *PLOS One, 7*(5), e36206.

feature of depression to return: Williams, M., Crane, C., Barnhofer, T., et al. (2006). Recurrence of suicidal ideation across depressive episodes. *Journal of Affective Disorders, 91,* 189–194; Williams, M., van der Does, W., Barnhofer, T., et al. (2008). Cognitive reactivity and suicidal ideation: Testing a differential activation theory of suicidality. *Cognitive Therapy & Research, 32,* 83–104.

PAGE 9

actively inhibit sensory pathways: Farb, N., & Segal, Z. (2024). *Better in every sense: How the new science of sensation can help you reclaim your life.* New York: Little, Brown Spark.

ONE. "Oh No, Here I Go Again": Why Unhappiness Won't Let Go

PAGE 19

depression tends to return: Birmaher, B., Arbelaez, C., & Brent, D. (2002). Course and outcome of child and adolescent major depressive disorder. *Child and Adolescent Psychiatric Clinics of North America, 11*(3), 619–637; Verduijn, J., Verhoeven, J., Milaneschi, Y., et al. (2017). Reconsidering the prognosis of major depressive disorder across diagnostic boundaries: Full recovery is the exception rather than the rule. *BMC Medicine, 15*(1), 215.

12 percent of men and 20 percent of women: Salk, R., Hyde, J., & Abramson, L. (2017). Gender differences in depression in representative national samples: Meta-analyses of diagnoses and symptoms. *Psychological Bulletin, 143*(8), 783–822.

Fifty percent of those: Kessler, R., Berglund, P., Demler, O., et al., (2003). The epidemiology of major depressive disorder: Results from the National Comorbidity Survey Replication (NCS-R). *Journal of the American Medical Association, 289,* 3095–3105; Zisook, S., Lesser, I., Stewart, J. W., et al. (2007). Effect of age at onset on the course of major depressive disorder. *American Journal of Psychiatry, 164*(10), 1539–1546; Williams, M., Barnhofer, T., Crane, C., et al. (2012). Pre-adult onset and patterns of suicidality in patients with a history of recurrent depression. *Journal of Affective Disorders, 138,* 173–179.

some 5 percent of the population: Global Health Data Exchange, Institute of Health Metrics and Evaluation. (2021). *Global burden of disease (GBD) results.* Retrieved from *https://vizhub.healthdata.org/gbd-results.*

15–39 percent of cases: Nierenberg, A. A. (2015). Residual symptoms in depression: Prevalence and impact. *Journal of Clinical Psychiatry, 76*(11), e1480.

22 percent of cases: Zajecka, J. M. (2013). Residual symptoms and relapse: Mood, cognitive symptoms, and sleep disturbances. *Journal of Clinical Psychiatry, 74*(Suppl 2), 9–13.

Each episode of depression: Solomon, D., Keller, M., Mueller, T., et al. (2000). Multiple recurrences of major depressive disorder. *American Journal of Psychiatry, 157,* 229–233.

Ten million people in the United States: Olfson, M., & Marcus, S. C. (2009). National patterns in antidepressant medication treatment. *Archives of General Psychiatry, 66*(8), 848–856. See also Kantor, E. D., Rehm, C. D., Haas, J. S., et al. (2015). Trends in prescription drug use among adults in the United States from 1999–2012. *Journal of the American Medical Association, 314*(17), 1818–1831.

PAGE 20

pioneering scientists like Aaron Beck: Beck, A. T. (1976). *Cognitive therapy and the emotional disorders.* New York: International Universities Press.

PAGE 22

feelings of low self-esteem and self-blame: Segal, Z., Kennedy, S., Gemar, M., et al. (2006). Cognitive reactivity to sad mood provocation and the prediction of depressive relapse. *Archives of General Psychiatry, 63*(7), 749–755.

PAGE 25

Automatic Thoughts: Hollon, S. D., & Kendall, P. (1980). Cognitive self-statements in depression: Development of an automatic thoughts questionnaire. *Cognitive Therapy and Research, 4,* 383–395. Copyright © 1980 Springer Nature. Reprinted by permission.

PAGE 27

aches and pains in the body: den Boeft, M., Twisk, J. W., Hoekstra, T., et al. (2016). Medically unexplained physical symptoms and work functioning over 2 years: Their association and the influence of depressive and anxiety disorders and job characteristics. *BMC Family Practice, 17,* 46.

psychologists asked people: Strack, F., Martin, L. L., & Stepper, S. (1988). Inhibiting and facilitating conditions of the human smile: A nonobtrusive test of the facial feedback hypothesis. *Journal of Personality and Social Psychology, 54,* 768–777.

PAGE 28

The inadvertent frowners: Laird, J. D. (1974). Self-attribution of emotion: The effects of expressive behaviour on the quality of emotional experience. *Journal of Personality and Social Psychology, 29,* 475–486.

a third study: See review in Gjelsvik, B., Lovic, D., & Williams, M. (2018). Embodied cognition and emotional disorders: Embodiment and abstraction in understanding depression. *Journal of Experimental Psychopathology, 9*(3), 1–41.

PAGE 30

The Exhaustion Funnel: Professor Åsberg used this figure in her talks to illustrate how exhaustion or "burnout" can progress—especially if people do not notice or do not take action when they start having symptoms. From an unpublished work by Marie Åsberg, 2004. Reprinted by permission.

TWO. **The Healing Power of Awareness: Making a Shift to Freedom**

PAGE 34

The most prominent are happiness, sadness: Ekman, P., & Davidson, R. J. (1995). *The nature of emotion: Fundamental questions.* New York: Oxford University Press. For an alternative view see Feldman Barrett, L. (2018). *How emotions are made.* Boston: Mariner Books.

PAGE 38

Memory researchers Duncan Godden and Alan Baddeley: Godden, D., & Baddeley, A. D. (1980). When does context influence recognition memory? *British Journal of Psychology, 71,* 99–104.

virtual reality environments: Shin, Y. S., Masís-Obando, R., Keshavarzian, N., et al. (2021). Context-dependent memory effects in two immersive virtual reality environments: On Mars and underwater. *Psychonomic Bulletin and Review, 28*(2), 574–582. See also Smith, S. M., & Vela, E. (2001). Environmental context-dependent memory: A review and meta-analysis. *Psychonomic Bulletin and Review, 8,* 203–220.

When we return to that mood: Eich, E. (1995). Searching for mood-dependent memory. *Psychological Science, 6,* 67–75.

PAGE 39
likely to be reactivated in the present: Cladder-Micus, M., van Aalderen, J., Donders, A., et al. (2018). Cognitive reactivity as outcome and working mechanism of mindfulness-based cognitive therapy for recurrently depressed patients in remission. *Cognition and Emotion, 32*(2), 371–378.

PAGE 43
when the doing mode started: Mason, T., Smith, K., Engwall, A., et al. (2019). Self-discrepancy theory as a transdiagnostic framework: A meta-analysis of self-discrepancy and psychopathology. *Psychological Bulletin, 145*(4), 372–389.

PAGE 44
hammer ourselves with more questions: These questions are taken from a measure of rumination by Susan Nolen-Hoeksema. See Nolen-Hoeksema, S. (2003). *Women who think too much.* New York: Holt.

PAGE 45
we believe that it will reveal: Papageorgiou, C., & Wells, A. (2001). Positive beliefs about depressive rumination: Development and preliminary validation of a self-report scale. *Behavior Therapy, 32,* 13–26; Watkins, E. R. (2008). Constructive and unconstructive repetitive thought. *Psychological Bulletin, 134,* 163–206.
rumination does exactly the opposite: Lyubomirsky, S., & Nolen-Hoeksema, S. (1995). Effects of self-focused rumination on negative thinking and interpersonal problem solving. *Journal of Personality and Social Psychology, 69,* 176–190.

THREE. Cultivating Mindfulness: A First Taste

PAGE 61
conducted an experiment: Simons, D. S., & Levin, D. T. (1998). Failure to detect changes to people during a real-world interaction. *Psychonomic Bulletin and Review, 5,* 644–649. See Simons, D., & Chabris, C. (2023). *Nobody's fool: Why we get taken in and what we can do about it.* New York: Basic Books.

PAGE 63
our full attention: This example is adapted from Nhat Hanh, T. (1975). *The miracle of mindfulness: A manual on meditation.* Boston: Beacon Press.

PAGE 64
"the hope of peace some day": Nhat Hanh, T. (1988). *The sun my heart.* Berkeley: Parallax Press (p. 125). Copyright © 2006 the Unified Buddhist Church. Reprinted

by permission of the Permissions Company on behalf of Parallax Press, Berkeley, California, www.parallax.org.

PAGE 66

The quality of mindfulness is not: Feldman, C. (2001). *The Buddhist path to simplicity: Spiritual practice for everyday life.* London: HarperCollins (p. 173). Copyright © 2009 Christina Feldman. Reprinted by permission of HarperCollins Publishers Ltd.

PAGE 67

reduces effort and makes the chosen activity easier: See Rosenberg, L., with Guy, D. (1998). *Breath by breath: The liberating practice of insight meditation.* Boston: Shambhala (p. 165).

FOUR. The Breath: Gateway to Awareness

PAGE 73

You cannot force the mind: This story is told by Ngakpa Chögyam: Chögyam, N. (1988). *Journey into vastness: A handbook of Tibetan meditation techniques.* Longmead, Shaftesbury, Dorset, U.K.: Element Books (pp. 28–32).

try not to think of a white bear: Garland, E., Brown, S., & Howard, M. (2016). Thought suppression as a mediator of the association between depressed mood and prescription opioid craving among chronic pain patients. *Journal of Behavioral Medicine, 39,* 128–138.

what we resist persists: Wegner, D. M. (2002). *The illusion of conscious will.* Cambridge, MA: MIT Press.

PAGE 74

keeping negative thinking at bay: Wenzlaff, R. M., & Bates, D. E. (1998). Unmasking a cognitive vulnerability to depression: How lapses in mental control reveal depressive thinking. *Journal of Personality and Social Psychology, 75,* 1559–1571.

more depressed than those who do not: Rude, S. S., Wenzlaff, R. M., Gibbs, B., et al. (2002). Negative processing biases predict subsequent depressive symptoms. *Cognition and Emotion, 16,* 423–440.

inhibiting the brain networks: Duncan, J. (2004). Selective attention in distributed brain systems. In M. I. Posner (Ed.), *Cognitive neuroscience of attention.* New York: Guilford Press (pp. 105–113); Tang, Y.-Y., & Posner, M. I. (2013). Tools of the trade: Theory and method in mindfulness neuroscience. *Social Cognitive and Affective Neuroscience, 8,* 118–120.

PAGE 82

cultivating a sense of appreciation: See Williams, M., & Penman, D. (2023). *Deeper mindfulness* (Chapter 6). New York: Balance. London: Piatkus.

FIVE. A Different Way of Knowing: Sidestepping the Ruminating Mind

PAGE 98

moving further away from physical experience: Allcott, H., Braghieri, L., Eichmeyer, S., et al. (2020). The welfare effects of social media. *American Economic Review*, 110(3), 629–676.

PAGE 110

learn to be present: Research in our Oxford lab by Catherine Crane and colleagues found that the more a person believed that their happiness depended on certain events turning out how they wanted, the less mindful they are. Crane, C., Barnhofer, T., Hargus, E., et al. (2010). The relationship between mindfulness and conditional goal setting in depressed patients. *British Journal of Clinical Psychology*, 42, 281–290.

SIX. Reconnecting with Our Feelings—Those We Like, Those We Don't Like, and Those We Don't Know We Have

PAGE 117

more than one hundred research studies: Hayes, S. C., Wilson, K. G., Gifford, E. V., et al. (1996). Experiential avoidance and behavioural disorders: A functional dimensional approach to diagnosis and treatment. *Journal of Consulting and Clinical Psychology*, 64, 1152–1168.

PAGE 119

messages of the internal barometer: Our recent research and practice has revealed several new ways to explore the "tipping point" moments and to bring more awareness, so dissolving the cascades of reactivity that might have followed. See Williams, M., & Penman, D. (2023). *Deeper mindfulness* (Chapter 7). New York: Balance.

way to tune in to body sensations: Farb, N., & Segal, Z. (2024). *Better in every sense: How the new science of sensation can help you reclaim your life*. New York: Little Brown.

PAGE 120

sadness activates the DMN: Farb, N. A. S., Desormeau, P., Anderson, A. K., et al. (2022). Static and treatment-responsive brain biomarkers of depression relapse vulnerability following prophylactic psychotherapy: Evidence from a randomized control trial. *NeuroImage Clinical*, 34, 102969.

following eight weeks of mindfulness-based cognitive therapy: The DMN also quiets down after an equivalent period of cognitive therapy (CT). This is not surprising as both CT and MBCT are known to be effective by the same mechanism— "decentering"—the ability to stand back from thoughts and see them as passing mental events.

PAGE 122

experiment with college students: Friedman, R. S., & Forster, J. (2001). The effects of promotion and prevention cues on creativity. *Journal of Personality and Social Psychology, 81,* 1001–1013.

flexibility in responding: There are also studies that have used different ways of inducing "approach" versus "avoidance" modes, for example by asking participants to pull a joystick toward them (approach) versus pushing it away (avoidance) and find similar effects. Phaf, R. H., Mohr, S. E., Rotteveel, M., et al. (2014). Approach, avoidance, and affect: A meta-analysis of approach-avoidance tendencies in manual reaction time tasks. *Frontiers of Psychology, 5,* 378.

PAGE 127

There's nothing extra we have to do: See Goldstein, J. (1994). *Insight meditation.* Boston: Shambhala. There are many talks by Joseph Goldstein available on *www. dharmaseed.com.*

PAGE 135

called the "Body Barometer": Bartley, T. (2017). *Mindfulness: A kindly approach to being with cancer.* Hoboken, NJ: Wiley-Blackwell (pp. 148–149). Copyright © 2017 Wiley-Blackwell. Reprinted by permission.

PAGE 136

The Bright Field: Thomas, R. S. (1995). *Collected poems 1945–1990.* London: Phoenix. Copyright © 2001 Orion Publishing Group (p. 302). Reprinted by permission.

SEVEN. Befriending Our Feelings

PAGE 139

How could we forget those ancient myths: Rilke, R. M. (1984). *Letters to a Young Poet.* Translated by Stephen Mitchell. New York: Modern Library (p. 27). Translation copyright © 1984 Stephen Mitchell, by permission of Random House, an imprint and division of Penguin Random House LLC. All rights reserved.

PAGE 148

brain pattern that underlies approach: Harmon-Jones, E., & Gable, P. A. (2018). On the role of asymmetric frontal cortical activity in approach and withdrawal motivation: An updated review of the evidence. *Psychophysiology, 55*(1), e12879.

PAGES 149–152

Amanda's Story: Segal, Z. V., Williams, J. M. G., & Teasdale, J. D. (2013). *Mindfulness-based cognitive therapy for depression, second edition.* New York: Guilford Press (pp. 282–284).

PAGE 155

"The Guest House": Barks, C., & Moyne, J. (trans.). (1997). *The essential Rumi*. San Francisco: Harper. Copyright © 1997 Coleman Barks (Maypop Books). Reprinted by permission.

EIGHT. Seeing Thoughts as Creations of the Mind

PAGE 161

is accessible to all of us if we dare to look: See Beck, A. T. (1976). *Cognitive therapy and the emotional disorders*. New York: International Universities Press.

PAGE 166

When we lose ourselves in thought: Goldstein, J. (1993). *Insight meditation*. Boston: Shambhala (pp. 59–60). See also Joseph Goldstein talks available on *www.dharmaseed.com*.

PAGE 169

Recognizing Automatic Negative Thoughts: Hollon, S. D., & Kendall, P. (1980). Cognitive self-statements in depression: Development of an Automatic Thoughts Questionnaire. *Cognitive Therapy and Research, 4*, 383–395. Copyright © 1980 Springer Nature. Reprinted by permission.

PAGE 173

The key to awakening: Brach, T. (2003). *Radical acceptance*. New York: Bantam Books (p. 188). See also talks by Tara Brach on *www.tarabrach.com* and *www.dharmaseed.com*.

PAGE 174

"It's okay not to like this": Saying "it's okay not to like this" is not saying that the thing that created the upset is okay. We are not saying it's okay to have deep depression or pain or trauma. Instead, we are saying that *it's natural not to like unpleasantness*. This allows the reactivity that surrounds the unpleasantness to drop away, so that it is not unwittingly exacerbated or maintained. See Williams, M., & Penman, D. (2023). *Deeper mindfulness* (Chapter 8). New York: Balance, & London: Piatkus.

NINE. Mindfulness in Everyday Life: Taking a Breathing Space

PAGE 177

Mindfulness is neither difficult: Feldman, C. (2001). *The Buddhist path to simplicity: Spiritual practice for everyday Life*. London: HarperCollins (p. 167). Copyright © 2009 Christina Feldman. Reprinted by permission of HarperCollins Publishers Ltd.

PAGE 196

rumination actively inhibits sensory processing: See Farb, N., & Segal, Z. (2024). *Better in every sense: How the new science of sensation can help you reclaim your life.* New York: Little, Brown Spark.

PAGE 199

engaging or reengaging in such activity: There are some very effective strategies for clinical depression that are based solely on engagement in activity. Dimidjian, S., Hollon, S. D., Dobson, K. S., et al. (2006). Randomized trial of behavioral activation, cognitive therapy, and anti-depressant medication in the acute treatment of adults with major depression. *Journal of Consulting and Clinical Psychology, 74,* 658–670; Patel, A., Weobong, B., Patel, V., et al. (2019). Psychological treatments for depression among women experiencing intimate partner violence: Findings from a randomized controlled trial for behavioral activation in Goa, India. *Archives of Women's Mental Health, 22*(6), 779–789.

PAGE 201

MBCT can help here too: National Institute for Health and Care Excellence. (2022). *Depression in adults: Treatment and management, NICE guideline* [NG 222]. *www. nice.org.uk/guidance/ng222.* See Strauss, C., Cavanagh, K., Oliver, A., et al. (2014). Mindfulness-based interventions for people diagnosed with a current episode of an anxiety or depressive disorder: A meta-analysis of randomised controlled trials. *PLOS One,* 9(4), e96110.

TEN. Fully Alive: Freeing Yourself from Chronic Unhappiness

PAGE 207

People say that what we're all seeking: Campbell, J., with Moyers, B. (1988). *The power of myth.* New York: Bantam Doubleday (p. 5).

PAGES 207–208

Arnold Lobel recounts a day in the life of Toad: Lobel, A. (1972). A List. In *Frog and Toad Together.* London: HarperCollins (pp. 4–17).

PAGE 210

I've been in this [prison] for six months now: These comments are from inmates of a Category B remand prison in the United Kingdom who were offered an eight-week mindfulness program by Andy Phee, Mark Williams, and Deborah Murphy, based on MBCT and the Peace in a Frantic World program.

Our theories, our research, and the stories: See Teasdale, J. (2022). *What happens in mindfulness.* New York: Guilford Press.

PAGE 218

Thich Nhat Hanh, a renowned: Nhat Hanh, T. (1991). *The sun my heart.* London: Rider (pp. 18, 23).

PAGE 219

Five steps for practicing mindfulness throughout the day: Rosenberg, L. (1998). *Breath by breath.* Boston: Shambhala (pp. 168–170).

PAGES 221–222

Everyday Mindfulness: Adapted from Madeline Klyne, Stress Reduction Clinic, University of Massachusetts Medical Center.

PAGE 223

Love after Love: Walcott, D. (2014). In *The poetry of Derek Walcott 1948–2013.* New York: Farrar, Straus & Giroux (p. 328). Copyright © 2014 Derek Walcott. Reprinted by permission of Farrar, Straus and Giroux. All rights reserved. Reprinted by permission of Faber and Faber Ltd. (U.K. and Commonwealth rights).

ELEVEN. Bringing It All Together: Weaving the Mindfulness Program into Your Life

PAGES 232–233

Pleasant Events Calendar: Modified from Kabat-Zinn, J. (1990). *Full catastrophe living.* New York: Hyperion.

PAGES 235–236

Unpleasant Events Calendar: Modified from Kabat-Zinn, J. (1990). *Full catastrophe living.* New York: Hyperion.

Index

Note. *f* following a page number indicates a figure.

About the Authors

Mark Williams, DPhil, is Professor of Clinical Psychology Emeritus at the University of Oxford Department of Psychiatry, where he was Founding Director of the Oxford Mindfulness Centre. He collaborated with John Teasdale and Zindel Segal in developing mindfulness-based cognitive therapy (MBCT) to prevent relapse and recurrence in major depression; together, they coauthored *Mindfulness-Based Cognitive Therapy for Depression, Second Edition* (for mental health professionals), as well as the self-help guide *The Mindful Way Workbook*. Dr. Williams continues to train mindfulness teachers internationally.

John Teasdale, PhD, held a Special Scientific Appointment with the United Kingdom Medical Research Council's Cognition and Brain Sciences Unit in Cambridge. He is a Fellow of the British Academy and the Academy of Medical Sciences. Since retiring, Dr. Teasdale has taught mindfulness and insight meditation internationally. He has continued to seek a psychological understanding of the wider implications of mindfulness and meditation for enhancing our way of being, and is the author of *What Happens in Mindfulness: Inner Awakening and Embodied Cognition.*

Zindel Segal, PhD, is Distinguished Professor of Psychology in Mood Disorders at the University of Toronto–Scarborough. Dr. Segal has conducted influential research into the psychological processes that make certain people more vulnerable than others to developing depression and experiencing recurrent episodes. He actively advocates for the relevance of mindfulness-based clinical care in psychiatry and mental health.

Jon Kabat-Zinn, PhD, is Professor of Medicine Emeritus at the University of Massachusetts Medical School, where he founded the Center for Mindfulness in Medicine, Health Care, and Society and the world-renowned Mindfulness-Based Stress Reduction program. Dr. Kabat-Zinn is the author of 15 books. His work and that of his colleagues around the world has contributed to the growing movement of mindfulness in mainstream society and in medicine, health care, psychology, and neuroscience. He teaches and conducts mindfulness retreats worldwide.

List of Audio Tracks